DO YOU HAVE THE NEW VIDEO?

Yes! There is a new video, available in either DVD or VHS format, that presents all 72 dialogues in this book. This totally revised supporting video with new contemporary characters effectively demonstrates all of the conversations and important structures — bringing life to the signs in the text. This video can be packaged with the text in either DVD or VHS format for a special discount.

Now you can study American Sign Language (ASL) in your own home by watching professional Deaf actors sign each sentence in a natural way. These fluent ASL users also model facial expressions and conversational gestures appropriate to ASL. By studying their use of ASL, you will be on your way to signing ASL fluently!

Order your video now! Cut this page on the dotted line, fill out the order form below, and mail to:

Pearson Education
Order Department
Box 11071
Des Moines, IA 50336

Or call 1-800-666-9433 to receive your video quickly.
You can also fax your order form to 1-800-835-5327.

Yes, I would like to order a copy of the video. Please send me:

Quantity:

_____ Book and Video Package (VHS format)
(includes both Learning American Sign Language, Second Edition by Tom Humphries and Carol Padden, and Video) (ISBN 0-205-40762-5) $104.99 **← Special Package Price!**

_____ Book and Video Package (DVD format)
(includes both Learning American Sign Language, Second Edition by Tom Humphries and Carol Padden, and Video) (ISBN 0-205-45391-0) $104.99 **← Special Package Price!**

_____ VHS alone (ISBN 0-205-27554-0) $61.99

_____ DVD alone (ISBN 0-205-45342-2) $61.99

_____ Book alone (ISBN 0-205-27553-2) $59.99

Prices subject to change without notice.

Name _____

Street Address _____

City _____

State _____ Zip Code _____

Signature _____

You will be billed for the total amount plus shipping and handling.
*If you decide you do not want the book or video, please return it **unopened** for a full refund.*

Learning ASL
American Sign Language

Levels I & II
Beginning & Intermediate

Second Edition

Tom Humphries
University of California, San Diego

Carol Padden
University of California, San Diego

Illustrations by
Rob Hills
Peggy Lott
Daniel W. Renner

PEARSON

Boston   New York   San Francisco
Mexico City   Montreal   Toronto   London   Madrid   Munich   Paris
Hong Kong   Singapore   Tokyo   Cape Town   Sydney

Executive Editor:	Stephen Dragin
Marketing Manager:	Tara Whorf
Production Administrator:	Susan Brown
Text Designer:	Máximo, Inc.
Formatting/Page Layout:	Máximo, Inc.
Composition Buyer:	Linda Cox
Manufacturing Buyer:	Andrew Turso

For related titles and support materials, visit our online catalog at www.ablongmon.com.

Library of Congress Cataloging-in-Publications Data

Humphries, Tom (Tom L.)
    Learning American sign language : levels I & II, beginning & intermediate / Tom Humphries, Carol Padden; illustrations by Rob Hills, Daniel W. Renner, Peggy Swartzel-Lott.
      p. cm.
      Includes index.
      ISBN 0-205-27553-2
      1. American Sign Language.   I. Padden, Carol.   II. Title.
HV2474.H862 2004
419'.7--dc21   2003044411

Printed in the United States of America
8 2019

CONTENTS

CONTENTS

Language Notes

CONTENTS

Culture Notes

To the Student

ou are now beginning to learn American Sign Language (ASL), the sign language used by Deaf people in the United States and parts of Canada. It is important to note that you are learning *American* Sign Language because there are many sign languages throughout the world that differ in structure and vocabulary from one another. As you learn about ASL in this book, you will also be learning about the culture of Deaf people in the United States.

Learning American Sign Language is structured to help you learn American Sign Language by presenting the vocabulary and sentences needed to communicate in common life situations. The sentence structures you need to learn are shown in context—that is, the grammar and vocabulary are tied together in some meaningful communicative situation. Notes discuss particular structures and rules that help you to master this language as well as give you cultural information for your interaction with Deaf American Sign Language users.

You should be aware that this book is not intended to be self-instructional. No book can be truly self-instructional when the objective is to learn a language that uses gesture and vision. However, the illustrations and exercises in this book will help you to recall and practice what your teacher has presented to you in class or what you have seen on practice videos. This book serves a purpose for which textbooks are ideally suited: to be a resource and reference for your ongoing study when no model of American Sign Language is present to demonstrate the language to you.

As with any other language, the amount of exposure you have to functional use of this language will help determine the speed at which you master it. Realistically, American Sign Language cannot be learned in a few weeks. The vocabulary and structures presented in this book require two semesters or three quarters of study. However, your fluency will depend on the number of class hours and the amount of interaction with users of this language that you have during your time of study.

The units of this book have a simple design. Each unit has a topic and is divided into subtopics. Each subtopic has a short dialogue that presents you with the structures and vocabulary of a real communicative situation. Key structures on which you should focus are selected from these dialogues and illustrated; some are discussed in short notes. Each unit has exercises that allow you to practice these useful structures. And finally, in each unit, there is a vocabulary list that is organized in categories for more effective study.

There are a few things you need to know to use this book. English translations of the American Sign Language sentences and vocabulary are given to help you understand the ranges of meaning for signs, but selecting exactly equivalent translations is very difficult, as often a change in the situational context will produce a different translation. Your teacher will be able to offer alternative translations that are equally suitable. Translations cannot be done on a "one word for one sign" basis. Sometimes a single sign requires several English words to translate it adequately or, conversely, a single English word requires several signs.

Signs are illustrated and labeled with capitalized English words. For example, the sign translated as "tree" is labeled TREE. This is a common way to label signs because there is no other widely accepted system for representing signs in print. The shortcoming of this system is that many signs do have multiple meanings or a wider range of meaning than the one- or two-word label assigned to it. Therefore, you should try to be aware of the full range of meaning of a sign rather than just that represented by the English label. In some places, signs that look exactly alike are assigned different labels because to assign them the same label would be confusing to you. Although using these English labels to represent signs may be a bit confusing at times, you should become accustomed to this convention and it will be less distracting.

As previously mentioned, sometimes a single sign requires a two- or three-word label. When this is done, the words are joined by hyphens as in NOT-YET. These two words joined by a hyphen represent just one sign. Hyphens are also used to join letters that represent fingerspelling used by American Sign Language users. Fingerspelling is a system of hand configurations that represent letters of the alphabet that are formed to spell out names or words. Therefore, J-O-H-N represents the fingerspelled letters of the name "John."

Other symbols are explained as they appear in the units. Your teacher will also be able to explain what these symbols represent. You will become used to them after a while.

On the inside front and back covers, you will find the fingerspelling and numbers system used in ASL. At the end of this book you will find a vocabulary index that will help you to find illustrations of signs in the text. You will find English translations of the ASL dialogues at the end of the book as well.

Acknowledgments

Writing and producing an ASL text is deceptively complex. We owe thanks to many people who contributed to the preparation of this book. Putting a visual language on the page so that it is useful to students is a challenge for authors, illustrators, and publisher. We are grateful to the sign models for posing for the many illustrations in this book: Lucinda O'Grady Batch, Monique Holt, Margarita Adams, Freda Norman, Donald Padden, Agnes Padden, John T. Reid, David Rivera, and Billy Seago. The illustrators: Rob Hills, Peggy Lott, and Danny Renner, with the help of Máximo Escobedo, brought the signs in this book to life. Monique Holt, Freda Norman, David Rivera, and Billy Seago deserve an extra round of thanks for performing in the accompanying video. Carlene Pederson spent hours checking and verifying the dialogues and sentences in this book against her wonderful intuition for the language. Susan Brown of Allyn & Bacon very ably coordinated the composition and preparation of the copy for publication and kept us and the book together and on schedule.

Sign Models

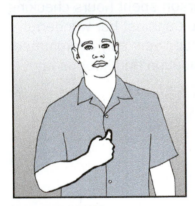

FREDA NORMAN

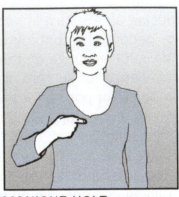

MONIQUE HOLT

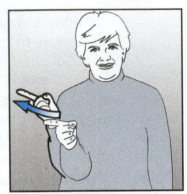

AGNES PADDEN

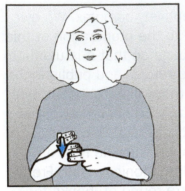

DAVID RIVERA

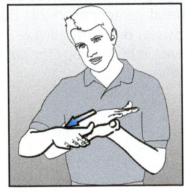

BILLY SEAGO

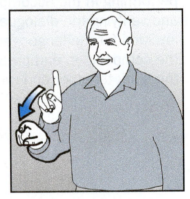

DONALD PADDEN

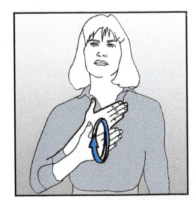

LUCINDA O'GRADY BATCH

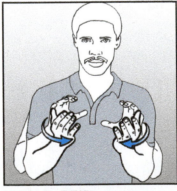

JOHN T. REID

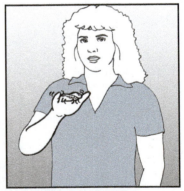

MARGARITA ADAMS

UNIT 1

Introductions and Personal Information

In this unit you will introduce yourself and give and get personal information.

You will use different types of questions and affirmative and negative sentences. You will also see how pronouns are used at the beginning and end of sentences.

In the culture notes, you will learn about the custom for giving your name, what Deaf people call themselves in ASL, and the difference between questions that ask where you live and where you are from.

INTRODUCTIONS

```
                              ____whq____
Alex:  I DON'T KNOW WHO YOU. NAME YOU?
                              ___whq___
Lisa:  I NAME L-I-S-A B-E-N-E-S. NAME YOU?

Alex:  I NAME A-L-E-X J-O-N-E-S. NICE MEET-YOU.

Lisa:  NICE MEET-YOU.
```

Key Structures

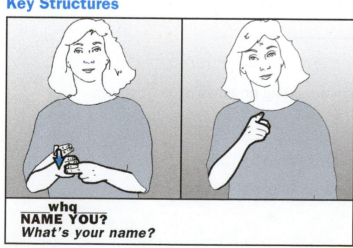

whq
NAME YOU?
What's your name?

Grammar Note

_____whq_____

Questions which ask for information such as NAME YOU? are signed with the eyebrows squeezed together and the head tilted forward (represented by the marker ___whq___). As with all question forms, the signer maintains eye contact with the person being asked the question.

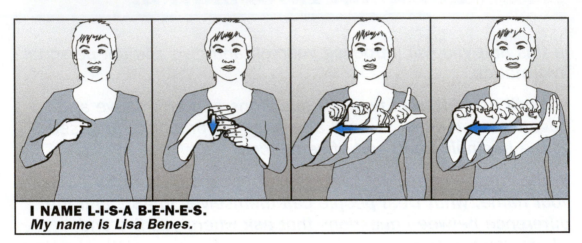

I NAME L-I-S-A B-E-N-E-S.
My name is Lisa Benes.

Culture Note

It is customary in first introductions, even casual ones, to offer your first and last name.

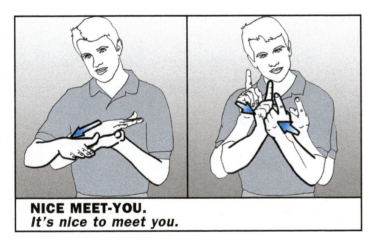

NICE MEET-YOU.
It's nice to meet you.

Exercise 1A

Introduce yourself to the classmate sitting on either side of you.

Prompt: Give your name.

　　　　　Ask for the other person's name.

　　　　　Express your pleasure at having met this person.

PERSONAL INFORMATION

                  _____q_____
Alex: YOU STUDENT YOU?

                    __q__
Lisa: YES. I STUDENT I. YOU?

Alex: NO. I NOT STUDENT I.

               _____q_____
Lisa: YOU DEAF YOU?

                    _____q_____
Alex: YES. I DEAF I. YOU HEARING YOU?

Lisa: YES. I HEARING I.

Key Structures

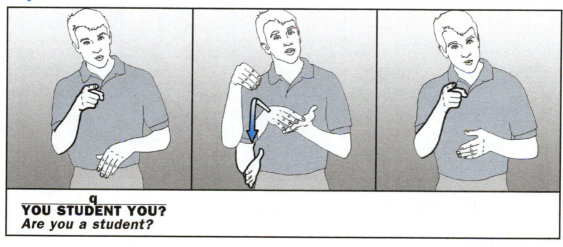

        q
YOU STUDENT YOU?
Are you a student?

Grammar Note

Questions which ask for a "yes" or "no" answer are signed with the eyebrows raised and the head tilted forward (represented by the marker ____q____). Remember to maintain eye contact with the person you are asking the question.

In questions such as these and in sentences such as I STUDENT I on the following page, the subject pronoun is sometimes repeated at the end of the sentence.

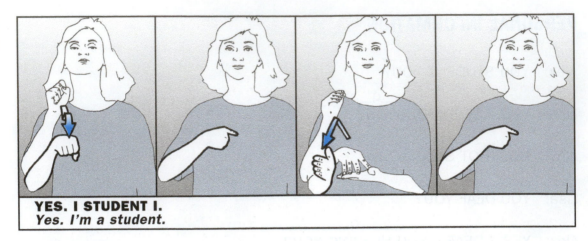

YES. I STUDENT I.
Yes. I'm a student.

Grammar Note

Simple affirmative sentences such as YES. I STUDENT I are accompanied by head nodding.

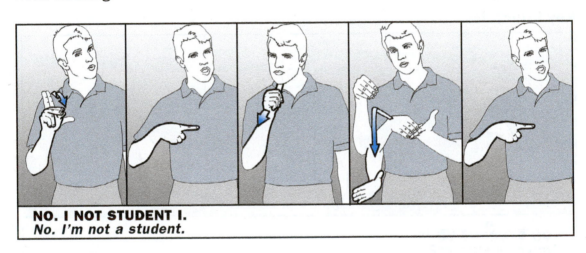

NO. I NOT STUDENT I.
No. I'm not a student.

Grammar Note

Simple negative sentences such as NO, I NOT STUDENT I are accompanied by head shaking.

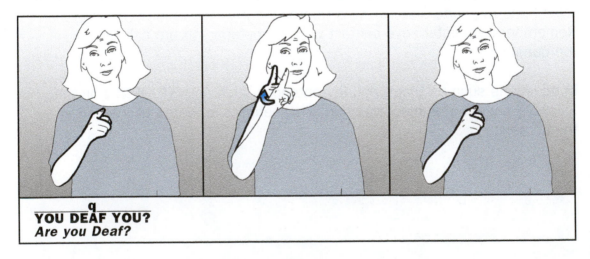

YOU DEAF YOU?
Are you Deaf?

Culture Note

DEAF is used in the above sentence to refer to the social and cultural identification of the person. DEAF is Deaf people's name for themselves. The sign may also be used to comment on hearing ability.

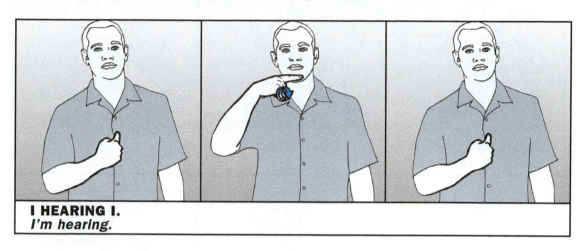

I HEARING I.
I'm hearing.

Exercise 1B

Complete this open dialogue.

Joe: Are you a student?
You: (Tell him you are a student and ask him if he is a student.)
Joe: No, I'm not a student. What's your name?
You: (Tell Joe your name and ask his name.)
Joe: My name is Joe.
You: (Ask Joe if he is Deaf.)
Joe: No, I'm not Deaf. Are you Deaf?
You: (Tell Joe if you are Deaf or hearing.)

MORE PERSONAL INFORMATION

```
          _____whq_____
Lisa:  WHERE FROM YOU?


Alex:  I FROM NEW-YORK.


Lisa:  I FROM CALIFORNIA.
          _____whq_____
Alex:  WHERE LIVE YOU?

              _____q_____
Lisa:  I LIVE S-D. YOU STUDENT YOU?


Alex:  NO. I YOUR TEACHER.
```

Key Structures

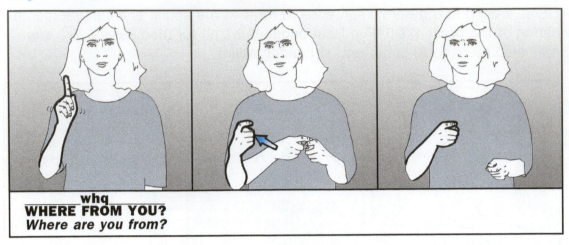

<u>whq</u>
WHERE FROM YOU?
Where are you from?

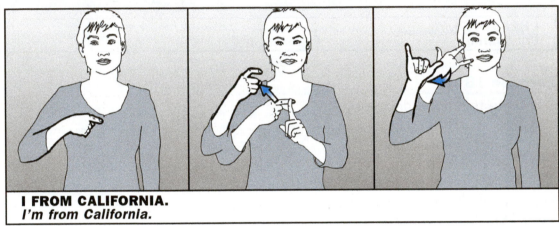

I FROM CALIFORNIA.
I'm from California.

Grammar Note

The sentence above is signed without repeating the subject pronoun at the end of the sentence. This variation is possible as are the following:

I STUDENT I.	I FROM CALIFORNIA I.	I NOT STUDENT I.
I STUDENT.	I FROM CALIFORNIA.	I NOT STUDENT.
STUDENT I.	FROM CALIFORNIA I.	NOT STUDENT I.

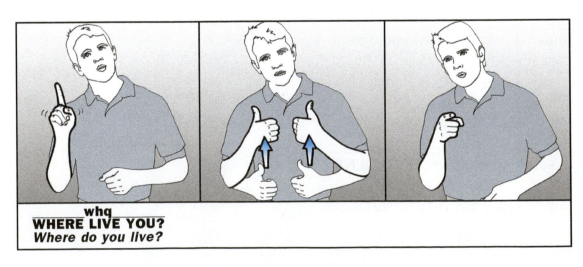

<u>whq</u>
WHERE LIVE YOU?
Where do you live?

Culture Note

_____whq_____
WHERE LIVE YOU? asks where you are currently living.

_____whq_____
WHERE FROM YOU? is different in that it usually asks where you are originally from. Among Deaf people it is used to ask which school for Deaf children you attended.

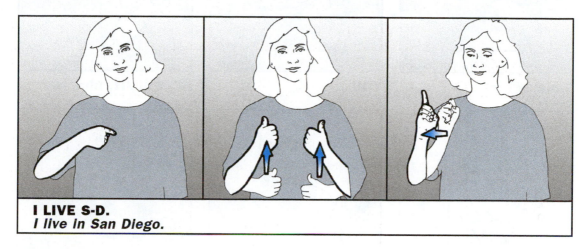

I LIVE S-D.
I live in San Diego.

Exercise 1C

Respond to the prompt:

1. What's your name?
2. Where are you from?
3. Are you a student or a teacher?
4. Where do you live?
5. Are you Deaf?
6. Ask the person next to you his/her name.
7. Ask the person next to you where he/she is from.
8. Ask the person next to you if he/she is a student or a teacher.
9. Ask the person next to you where he/she lives.
10. Ask the person next to you if he/she is Deaf.

VOCABULARY

▶ **Pronouns**

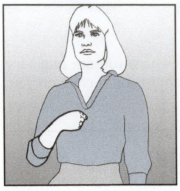

I, me

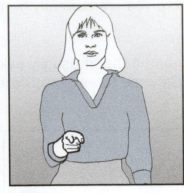

YOU

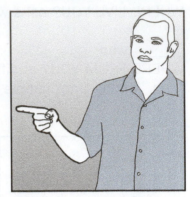

HE/SHE/IT, him/her

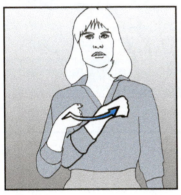

WE, us

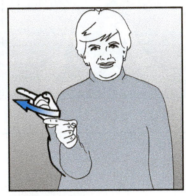

THEY, them

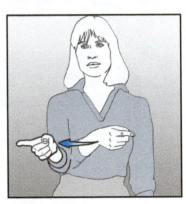

YOU–plural

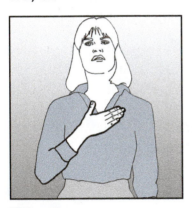

MY, mine

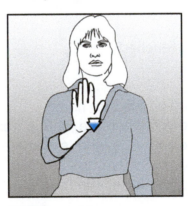

YOUR, yours

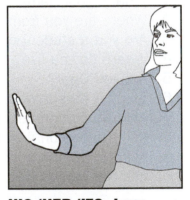

HIS/HER/ITS, hers

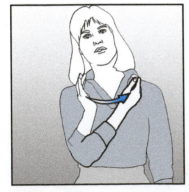

OUR, ours

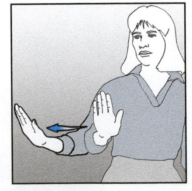

THEIR, theirs

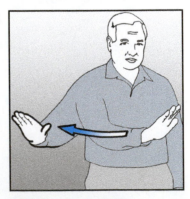

YOUR–pl., yours

▶ **Question Signs**   ▶ **People**

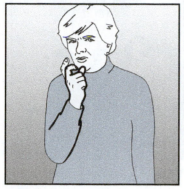

WHO

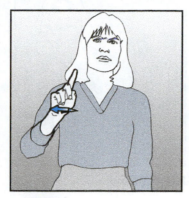

WHERE

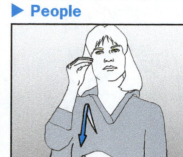

STUDENT

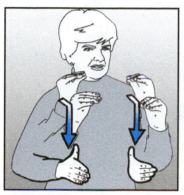

TEACHER, professor

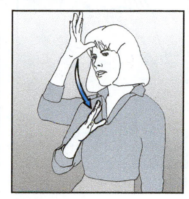

MAN

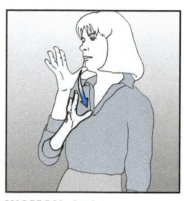

WOMAN, lady

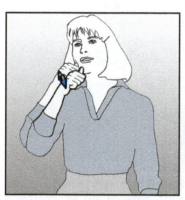

GIRL

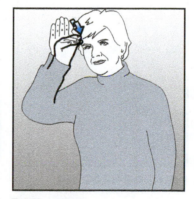

BOY, man

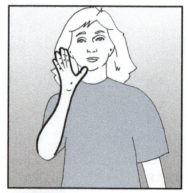

MOTHER

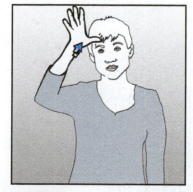

FATHER

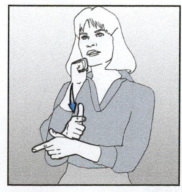

SISTER

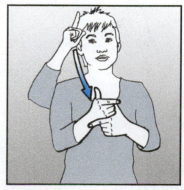

BROTHER

▶ **Places**

▶ **Other Vocabulary**

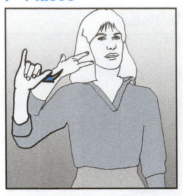

CALIFORNIA, gold

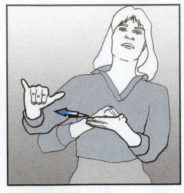

NEW-YORK

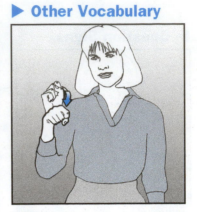

YES

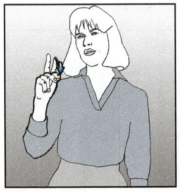

NO

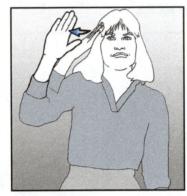

DON'T-KNOW

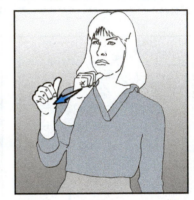

NOT

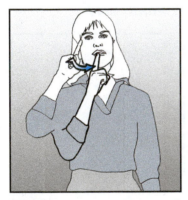

DEAF

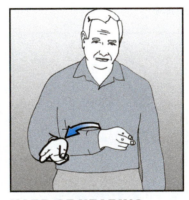

HARD-OF-HEARING

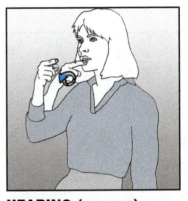

HEARING (person), say, speaking

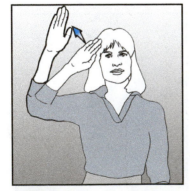

HELLO, hi

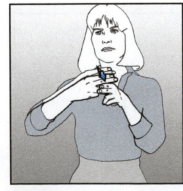

NAME

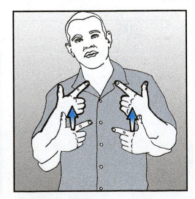

LIVE–1, life

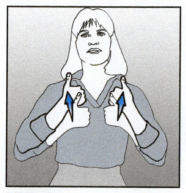

LIVE–2

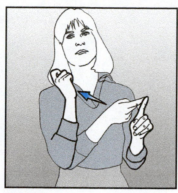

FROM

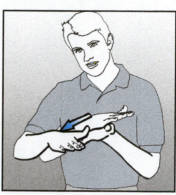

NICE, clean, pure

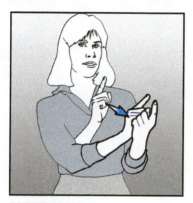

MEET-YOU

UNIT 2

Learning ASL

In this unit you will talk about being in an ASL class and how to show that you understand or ask for help.

You will answer questions by repeating the verb in the question. You will learn the two types of "there." You will use three different forms of questions that ask for information.

And you will learn the use of OH-I-SEE.

GOING TO CLASS

```
                    q
_____
```
Chris: TAKE-UP A-S-L CLASS YOU?

Lisa: YES, I TAKE-UP.

```
        whq
_____
```
Chris: WHICH CLASS?

Lisa: CLASS CALLED A-S-L ONE.

```
              whq
_____
```
Chris: SAME-AS-ME! WHERE CLASS?

Lisa: CLASS THERE COLLEGE.

Key Structures

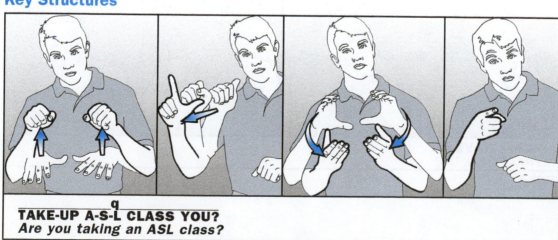

```
          q
_____
```
TAKE-UP A-S-L CLASS YOU?
Are you taking an ASL class?

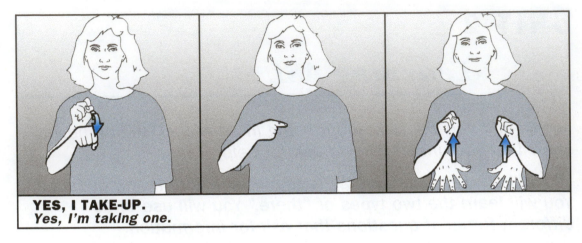

YES, I TAKE-UP.
Yes, I'm taking one.

Grammar Note

Questions which ask for a yes or no answer can be answered by repeating the verb from the question. Another example:

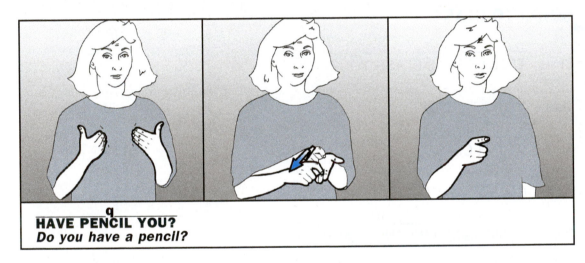

q
HAVE PENCIL YOU?
Do you have a pencil?

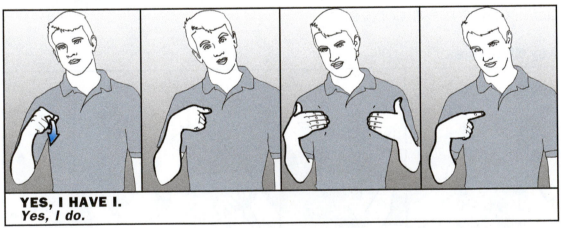

YES, I HAVE I.
Yes, I do.

2

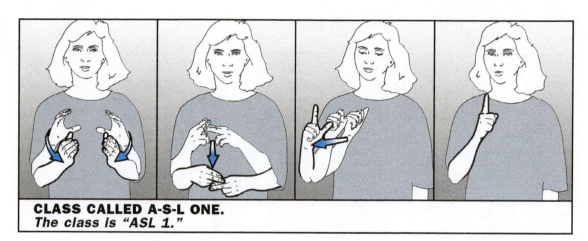

CLASS CALLED A-S-L ONE.
The class is "ASL 1."

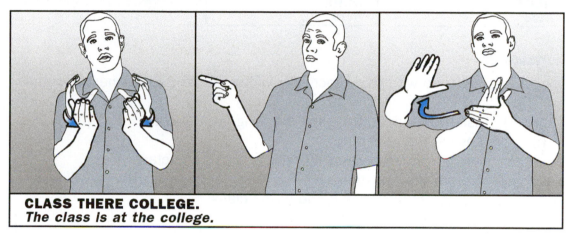

CLASS THERE COLLEGE.
The class is at the college.

Grammar Note

When the place is not in sight, the sign THERE is made in the approximate direction of the place as in the example above.

In another form of THERE, the specific location of an object is indicated and the signer looks directly at the object. Notice the short directional movement at the end of the sign in the following example:

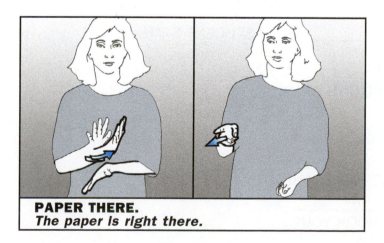

PAPER THERE.
The paper is right there.

There are two forms which mean "here."

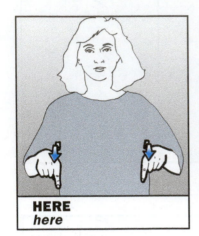

HERE
here

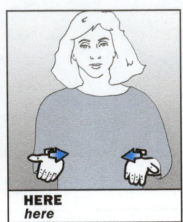

HERE
here

Exercise 2A

Repeat this dialogue with your teacher or with a student sitting next to you.

(Teacher)   Ask the student if he/she is taking an ASL class.
(You)   Answer the question.
(Teacher)   Ask the student where he/she is taking the class.
(You)   Answer the question.
(Teacher)   Ask the student the name of the class.
(You)   Answer the question.

Exercise 2B

Identify yourself and the student next to you until all of you have introduced each other. Follow the prompts:

(You)   I NAME _____.

                                                    _____q_____
               SHE NAME _____. NAME YOU?

(Other student) I NAME _____. I STUDENT SAME-AS-YOU.

OBJECTS IN THE CLASSROOM

          _____q_____
Chris: HAVE PENCIL YOU?

                  _____whq_____
Lisa: YES, I HAVE I. WHERE PAPER WHERE?

                _____q_____
Chris: PAPER THERE. HAVE BOOK YOU?

               _____whq_____
Lisa: NO, WHERE BOOK WHERE?

Key Structures

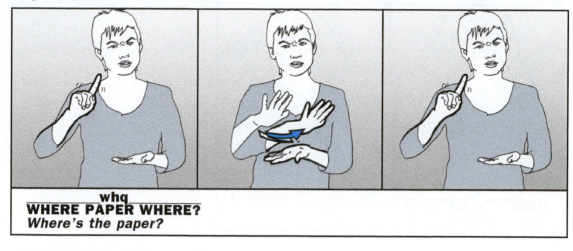

```
           whq
WHERE PAPER WHERE?
Where's the paper?
```

2

Grammar Note

In questions which ask for information such as:

```
_____whq_____
WHERE PAPER WHERE?
```

the following forms can also be used:

```
_____whq_____
WHERE PAPER?
_____whq_____
PAPER WHERE?
```

Exercise 2C

Ask the student next to you if he/she has the following items and wait for an answer.

1. paper
2. a pencil
3. a book

Ask the student next to you where these items are and wait for an answer.

SHOWING YOU UNDERSTAND AND ASKING FOR HELP

```
            q
```
Alex: UNDERSTAND YOU?

Lisa: NOT UNDERSTAND I. AGAIN PLEASE.

Alex: HERE CLASS A-S-L ONE.

Lisa: OH-I-SEE. UNDERSTAND I.

Key Structures

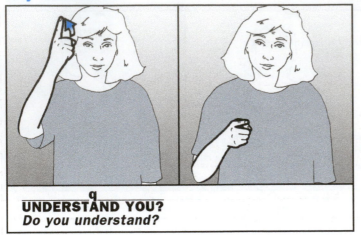

q
UNDERSTAND YOU?
Do you understand?

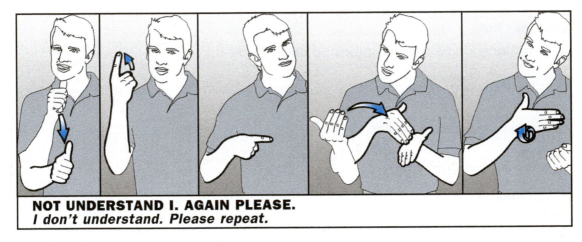

NOT UNDERSTAND I. AGAIN PLEASE.
I don't understand. Please repeat.

Note

Other ways to ask for help include:

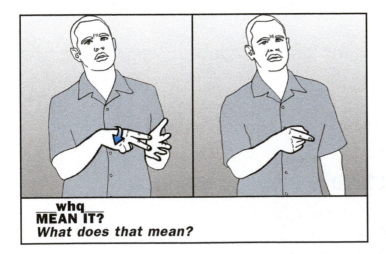

whq
MEAN IT?
What does that mean?

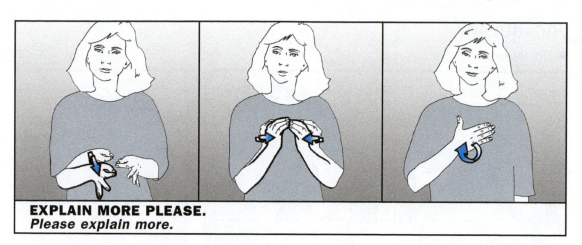

EXPLAIN MORE PLEASE.
Please explain more.

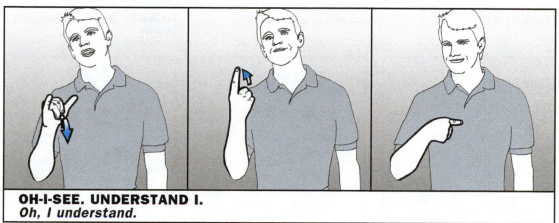

OH-I-SEE. UNDERSTAND I.
Oh, I understand.

Note

The sign OH-I-SEE can also be used alone to show that you understand or that you are following what is being said. It is *not* used for an affirmative response; the sign YES is used for that purpose.

Exercise 2D

Complete this open dialogue.

Kathy: My name is Kathy.
You: (Tell her you don't understand and ask her to repeat.)
Kathy: My name is Kathy. Do you understand?
You: (Tell her you understand and give her your name.)
Kathy: Is this the ASL class?
You: (Tell her that yes, this is the ASL class and ask if she is a student too.)
Kathy: Yes. Who's the teacher?
You: (Ask her what TEACHER means.)
Kathy: The teacher, who's the teacher?
You: (Tell her you understand.)

VOCABULARY

▶ **In Class**

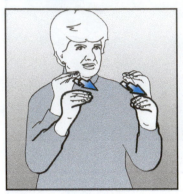

TEACH, educate

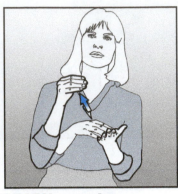

LEARN, acquire

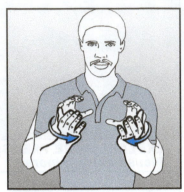

CLASS, group, category, team

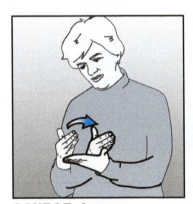

COURSE, lesson

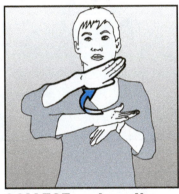

COLLEGE, university

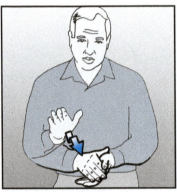

SCHOOL, academic

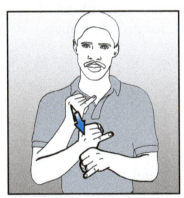

RESIDENTIAL-SCHOOL, school for the Deaf, institution, institute

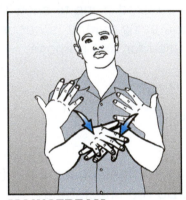

MAINSTREAM

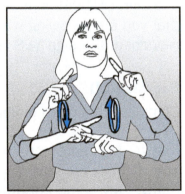

SIGN, sign language, signing

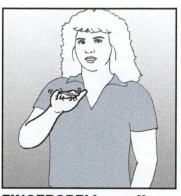

FINGERSPELL, spell

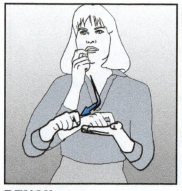

PENCIL, pen

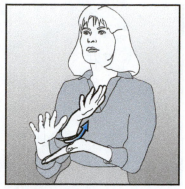

PAPER, page

▶ **Question Signs**

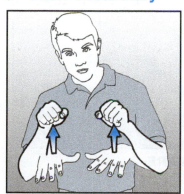

BOOK

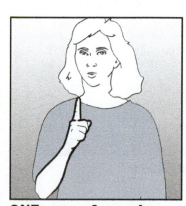

WHICH

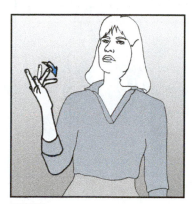

WHY

▶ **Other Vocabulary**

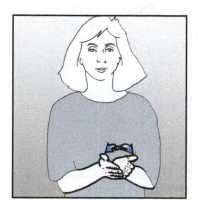

TAKE-UP, adopt

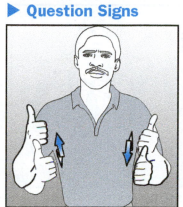

ONE, one of a series

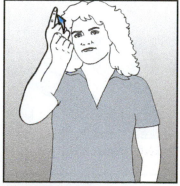

UNDERSTAND

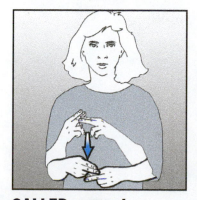

CALLED, named

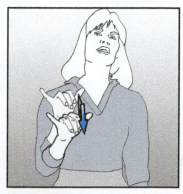

OH-I-SEE

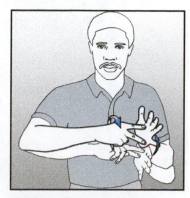

MEAN, meaning

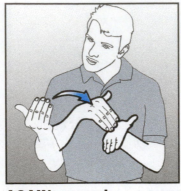

EXPLAIN, describe

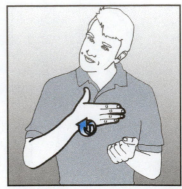

AGAIN, repeat

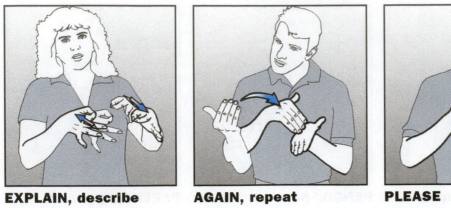

PLEASE

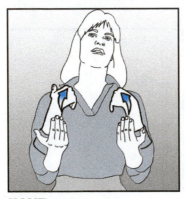

HAVE, own

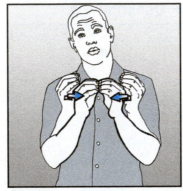

MORE

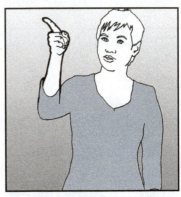

THERE (approximate)

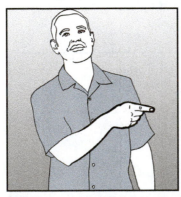

THERE (specific)

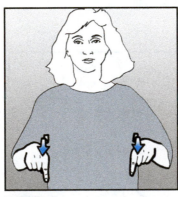

HERE–1

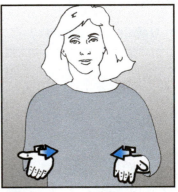

HERE–2

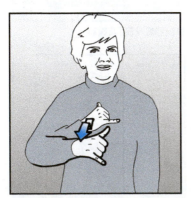

SAME-AS-ME/YOU

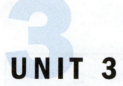

UNIT 3

Politeness

In this unit, you will use the language of politeness: how to ask politely and how to say thank you. You will also learn how to interrupt politely and how to apologize.

You will use verbs that change movement to show location or to indicate subject and object.

You will also learn what to do when walking between signers.

ASKING POLITELY

<table>
<tr><td></td><td>_____whq_____
Lisa: EXCUSE-ME. LIBRARY WHERE?</td></tr>
</table>

Lisa: EXCUSE-ME. LIBRARY WHERE?

Alex: I GO-THERE NOW. COME-ON ACCOMPANY.

Lisa: FINE. WAIT-ONE-MINUTE PLEASE. BOOK GET I.

Alex: O-K. I NOT HURRY I.

Key Structures

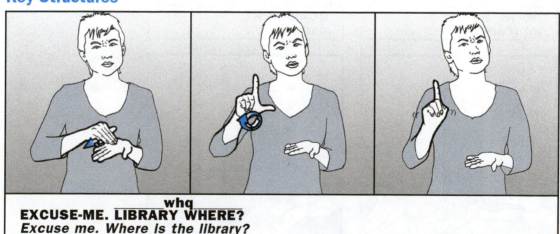

EXCUSE-ME. <u>LIBRARY WHERE?</u>
Excuse me. Where is the library?

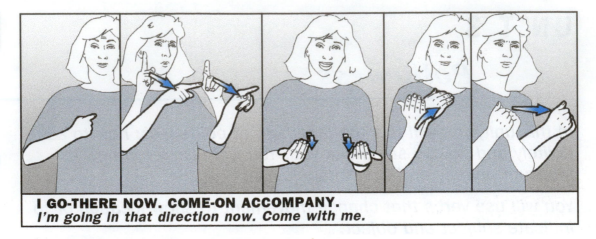

I GO-THERE NOW. COME-ON ACCOMPANY.
I'm going in that direction now. Come with me.

Grammar Note

Some verbs such as GO/COME, BRING/CARRY, and MOVE change the direction of their movement to show a change from one location to another as in GO-THERE above. The direction of the movement is from the first location to the second location. Some examples are:

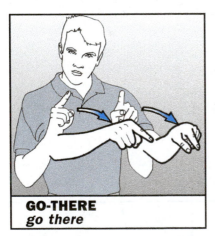

GO-THERE
go there

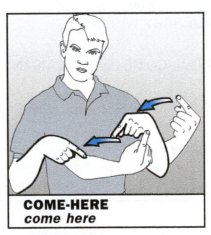

COME-HERE
come here

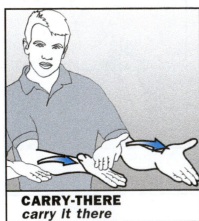

CARRY-THERE
carry it there

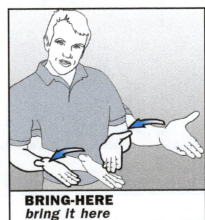

BRING-HERE
bring it here

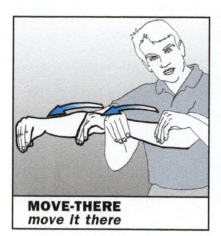

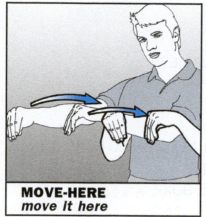

MOVE-THERE
move it there

MOVE-HERE
move it here

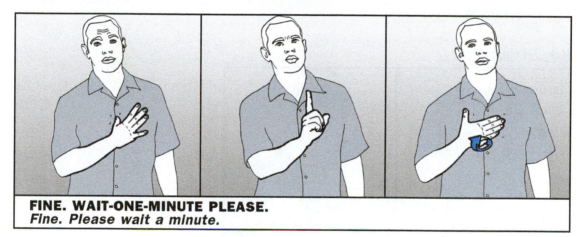

FINE. WAIT-ONE-MINUTE PLEASE.
Fine. Please wait a minute.

Exercise 3A

Tell the student next to you that you are going to the following places:

1. to the library
2. to class
3. to the college
4. to the bookstore
5. to the cafeteria

Then tell the student next to you to bring the following items to you:

1. box
2. paper
3. chair
4. television
5. book

THANKS

Pat: <u>_____q_____</u>
CAN YOU-HELP-ME?

Chris: <u>____whq____</u>
SURE. WHAT NEED?

Pat: THANK-YOU. I NEED BRING-HERE BOX.

Chris: <u>____whq_____</u>
SURE. WHERE BOX?

Pat: THANKS-A-LOT.

Key Structures

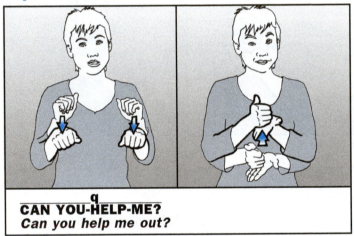

<u>_____q_____</u>
CAN YOU-HELP-ME?
Can you help me out?

Grammar Note

Some verbs change the direction of their movement to indicate the subject and object of the verb such as in YOU-HELP-ME above. The movement can be changed to show the following:

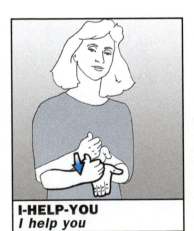

I-HELP-YOU
I help you

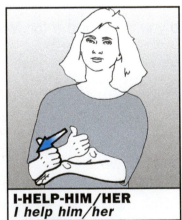

I-HELP-HIM/HER
I help him/her

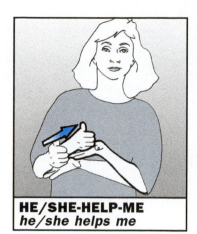

HE/SHE-HELP-ME
he/she helps me

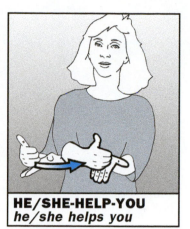

HE/SHE-HELP-YOU
he/she helps you

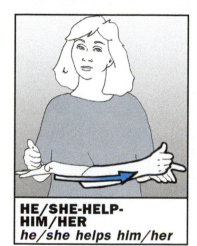

**HE/SHE-HELP-
HIM/HER**
he/she helps him/her

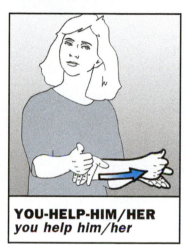

YOU-HELP-HIM/HER
you help him/her

Some other verbs that can do this are:

ASK	LOOK-AT	SEND
TELL	PAY	
SHOW	GIVE	

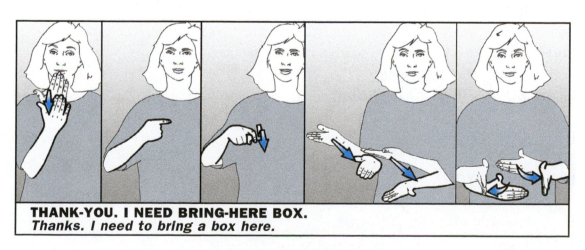

THANK-YOU. I NEED BRING-HERE BOX.
Thanks. I need to bring a box here.

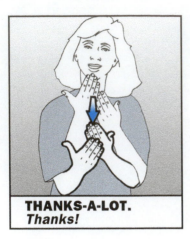

THANKS-A-LOT.
Thanks!

Exercise 3B

Tell the student next to you to:

1. send you a box
2. send another student a box
3. show you a book
4. show another student a book
5. ask another student his/her name
6. tell another student his/her name
7. give you a book
8. give another student a book
9. pay you
10. pay another student

INTERRUPTIONS AND APOLOGIES

Lisa: EXCUSE-ME.

       _whq__

Pat: WHAT?

               _____whq_____

Lisa: SORRY. RESTROOM WHERE?

Pat: DOWN-THERE.

Lisa: THANK-YOU.

Key Structures

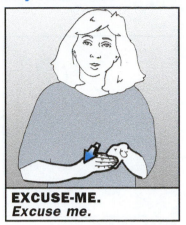

EXCUSE-ME.
Excuse me.

Culture Note

It is particularly important to say EXCUSE-ME if there is no way to reasonably avoid walking between two signers who are having a conversation.

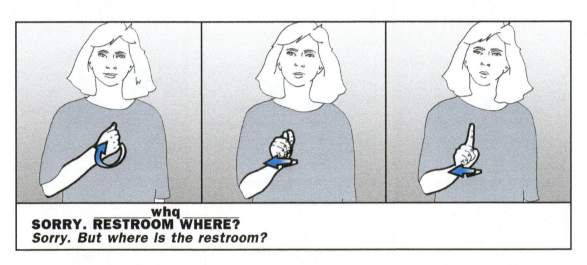

<u>whq</u>
SORRY. RESTROOM WHERE?
Sorry. But where is the restroom?

Exercise 3C

Interrupt the student next to you, apologize, and ask the following questions:

1. his/her name
2. where your sign language book is
3. where the restroom is
4. where the television is
5. where some paper is

VOCABULARY

▶ **Politeness**

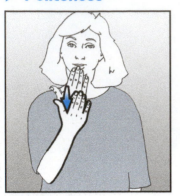

THANK-YOU

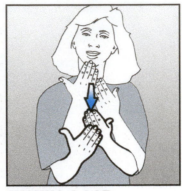

THANKS-A-LOT

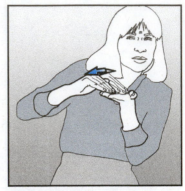

EXCUSE-ME, pardon-me

▶ **Items and Places at School**

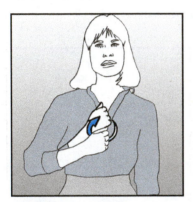

SORRY, apologize

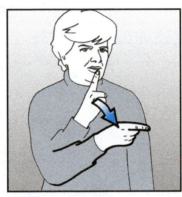

SURE, really, true

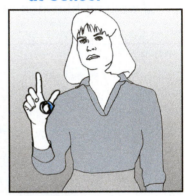

LIBRARY

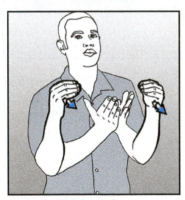

BOOKSTORE

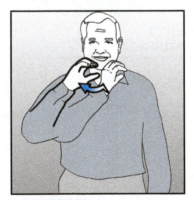

CAFETERIA

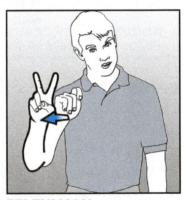

TELEVISION

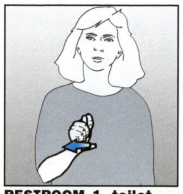

RESTROOM–1, toilet

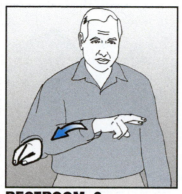

RESTROOM–2

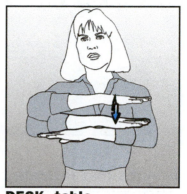

DESK, table

▶ **Verbs that Indicate Subject-Object**

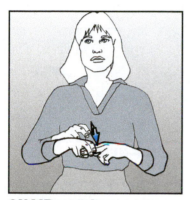

CHAIR, seat

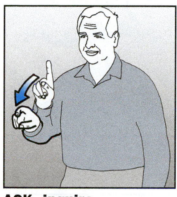

ASK, inquire

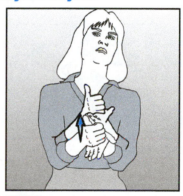

HELP

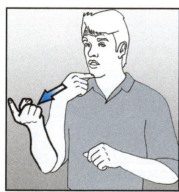

TELL

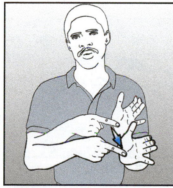

SHOW, demonstrate, example

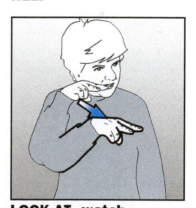

LOOK-AT, watch

3

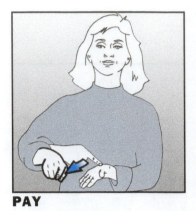

PAY

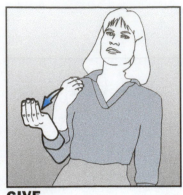

GIVE

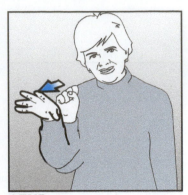

SEND

▶ **Verbs that Indicate Location**

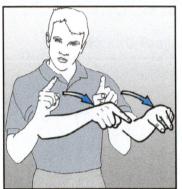

GO–THERE

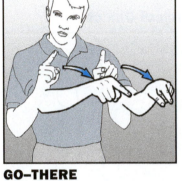

COME–HERE

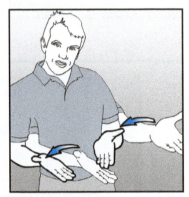

BRING–HERE

▶ **Other Vocabulary**

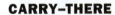

CARRY–THERE

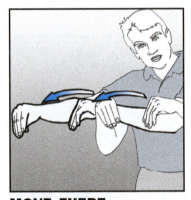

MOVE–THERE

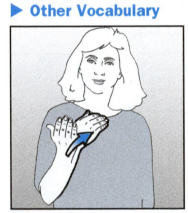

COME-ON

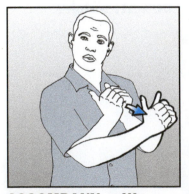

ACCOMPANY, with, together

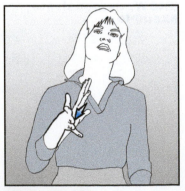

FINE, great!

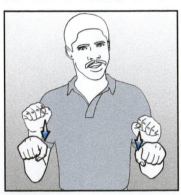

CAN

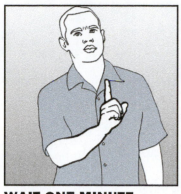

WAIT-ONE-MINUTE

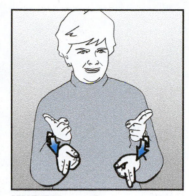

HURRY, rush

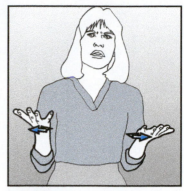

WHAT–1

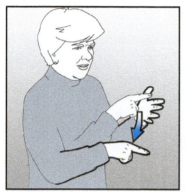

WHAT–2

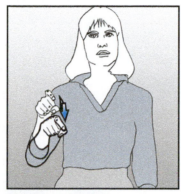

NEED, should

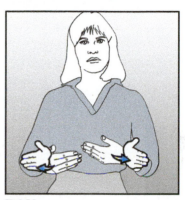

BOX

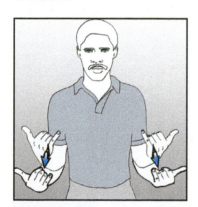

NOW, today, presently

3

UNIT 4

Descriptions

In this unit, you will learn about describing people: their physical appearance, their clothing, and their personalities and character.

You will ask what someone looks like and how to use adjectives describing hair, height, and weight. You will learn the position of descriptive adjectives in sentences. You will see how signs are altered to show detail such as the direction of stripes.

And, finally, you will learn about topicalization of subjects and objects.

4

PHYSICAL APPEARANCE

```
                        q
Chris: YOU KNOW MY TEACHER YOU?

                        ___whq___
Pat:   NO, DON'T-KNOW. LOOK^LIKE?
```

Chris: HAIR SHOULDER-LENGTH BLACK, EYES BROWN.

Pat: EXPLAIN MORE.

Chris: TALL, THIN.

Pat: OH-I-SEE, I KNOW WHO.

Key Structures

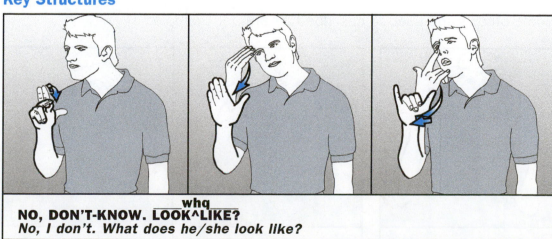

NO, DON'T-KNOW. LOOK^LIKE?
No, I don't. What does he/she look like?

Grammar Note

_____whq_____

Remember that the question LOOK^LIKE? is made like other questions asking for information, with eyebrows squeezed together and the head tilted slightly forward.

The mark, ^, indicates that the sign LOOK^LIKE is a contraction of two signs, APPEARANCE and SAME, in which the movement is made like one sign. Compare below:

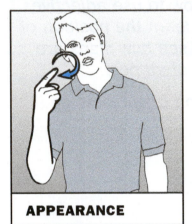

APPEARANCE

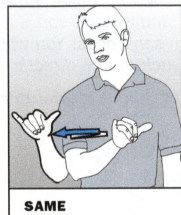

SAME

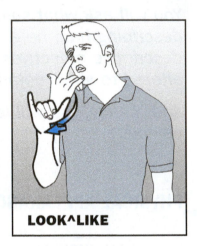

LOOK^LIKE

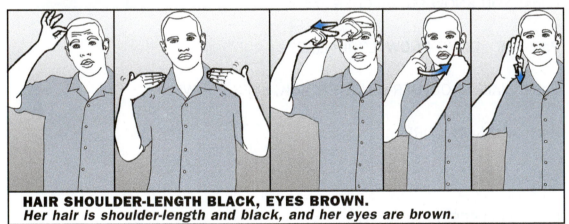

HAIR SHOULDER-LENGTH BLACK, EYES BROWN.
Her hair is shoulder-length and black, and her eyes are brown.

Grammar Note

Some other signs used to describe hair are, for example:

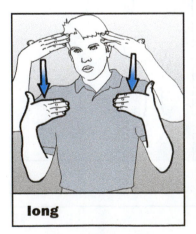

long

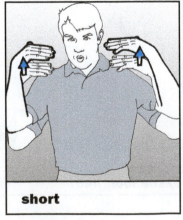

short

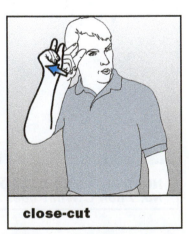

close-cut

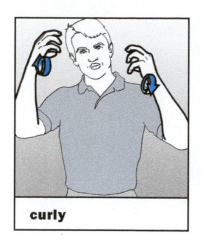

curly

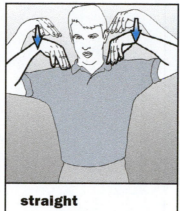

straight

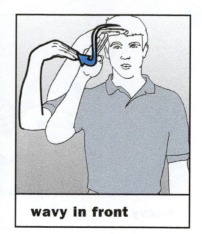

wavy in front

4

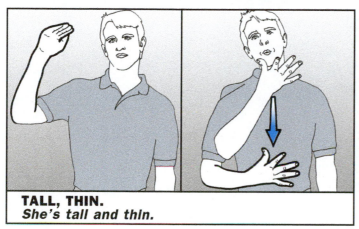

TALL, THIN.
She's tall and thin.

Grammar Note

Some other signs used to describe height and weight are:

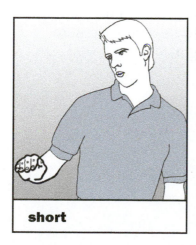

short

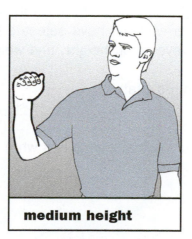

medium height

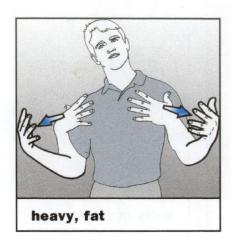

heavy, fat

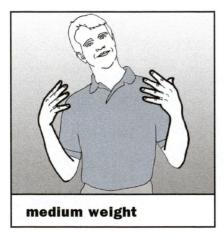

medium weight

Exercise 4A

Working in pairs and taking turns, describe the following people to each other. Don't tell your partner who you have selected to describe. Be sure to give hairstyle and color, eye color, height, and weight.

1. the President of the United States
2. your mother
3. your father
4. a movie star (see if your partner can guess who)
5. Santa Claus

CLOTHING

```
                          _____q_____
```
Pat: SEE WOMAN THERE, RED DRESS?

```
       __whq__
```
Alex: WHICH?

Pat: THERE STRIPES (vertical), LONG-SKIRT.

```
       _____q_____
```
Alex: YOU MEAN WHITE HAT?

Pat: THAT-ONE.

Key Structures

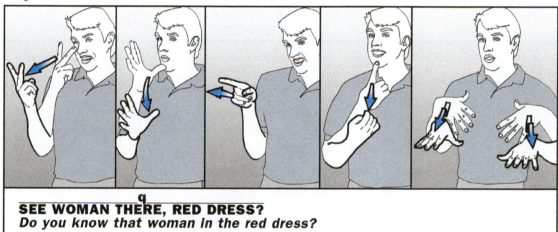

```
              q
```
SEE WOMAN THERE, RED DRESS?
Do you know that woman in the red dress?

Grammar Note

Colors (RED, BLUE, etc.) may appear before or after a noun. The sentence above could be signed as follows:

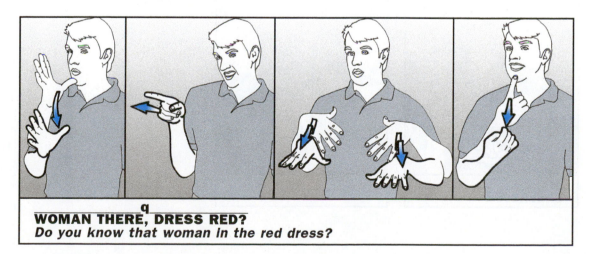

```
              q
```
WOMAN THERE, DRESS RED?
Do you know that woman in the red dress?

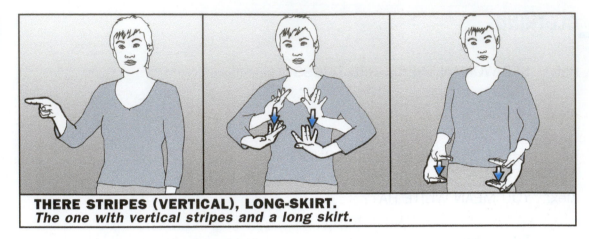

THERE STRIPES (VERTICAL), LONG-SKIRT.
The one with vertical stripes and a long skirt.

Grammar Note

Certain descriptive signs can be altered to show specific detail, for example, the direction of stripes or the length of a dress or skirt:

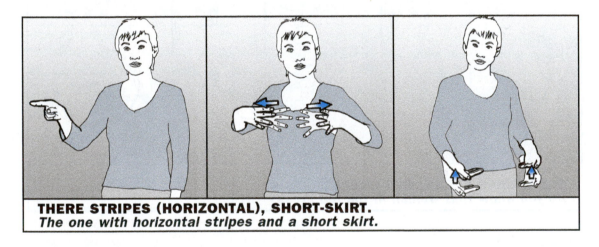

THERE STRIPES (HORIZONTAL), SHORT-SKIRT.
The one with horizontal stripes and a short skirt.

Some other signs for describing clothing are:

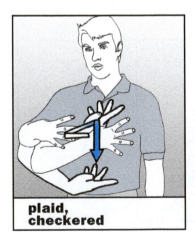

plaid, checkered

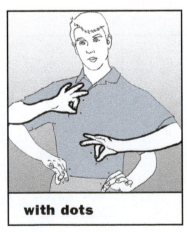

with dots

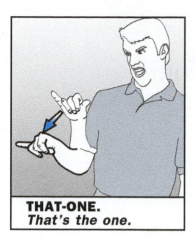

THAT-ONE.
That's the one.

Exercise 4B

Describe the clothing in the following pictures:

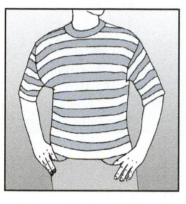

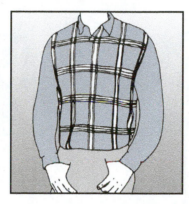

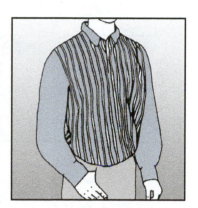

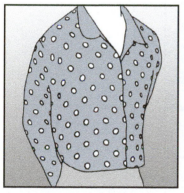

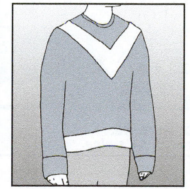

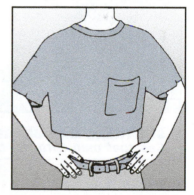

4

PERSONALITY AND CHARACTER

Chris: SEE THERE MAN BEARD, NICE HE. YOU KNOW HE?

_____t_____   _____q_____

Alex: NOT-YET MEET-HIM.

Chris: HE FRIENDLY. MAN THERE ARROGANT.

_____t_____

Alex: I KNOW HE. RIGHT YOU. ARROGANT HE.

Key Structures

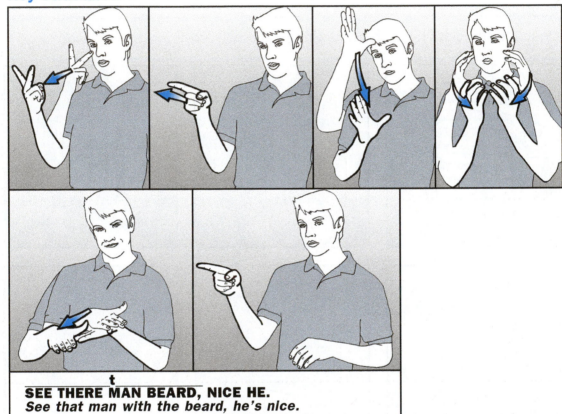

SEE THERE MAN BEARD, NICE HE.

_____t_____

See that man with the beard, he's nice.

Grammar Note

The subject or object of a sentence can be introduced first as the topic of the sentence and followed by a comment as in the sentence above. To show a topic use raised eyebrows while signing the topic. (The raised eyebrows are indicated here by the topic marker _____t_____ above.) Other examples:

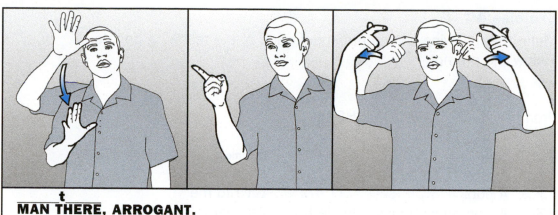

$\overline{\text{MAN}\ \overset{t}{\overline{\text{THERE}}}}$, ARROGANT.
That man, he's arrogant.

4

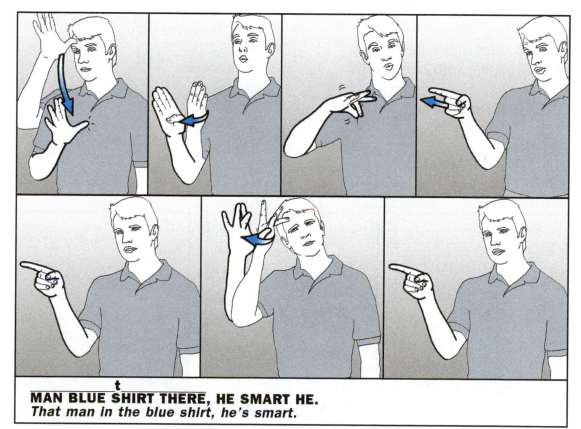

$\overline{\text{MAN BLUE}\ \overset{t}{\overline{\text{SHIRT THERE}}}}$, HE SMART HE.
That man in the blue shirt, he's smart.

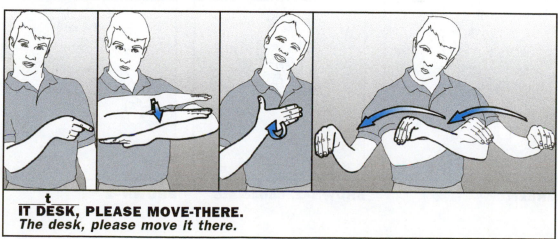

$\overline{\text{IT}\ \overset{t}{\overline{\text{DESK}}}}$, PLEASE MOVE-THERE.
The desk, please move it there.

Exercise 4C

Make the following comments about each of the following people.
Follow the prompt.

```
            t
_____
```
Prompt: MAN BLUE COAT, HE NICE.

	Topic	Comment
1.	A man in striped pants	Friendly
2.	A book	Give to me
3.	A woman with long, blonde hair	Ask her to come here
4.	A man in a green coat	Arrogant
5.	A girl	Smart
6.	A boy with curly hair	Tell him to come here
7.	A man with a beard	Heavy
8.	Teacher with blue shirt	Good teacher
9.	A coat with red dots	Bring it here
10.	A heavyset man	Pay him

VOCABULARY

▶ **Colors**

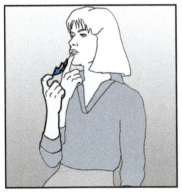

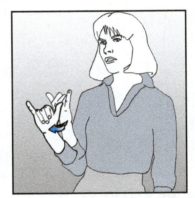

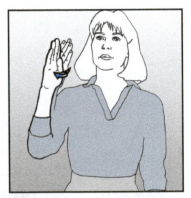

RED   **YELLOW**   **BLUE**

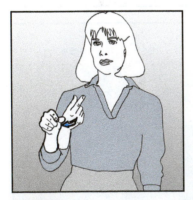

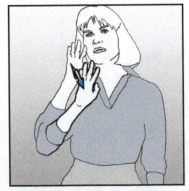

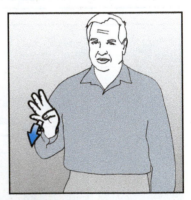

GREEN   **BROWN–1, chocolate**   **BROWN–2**

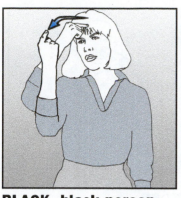

BLACK, black person

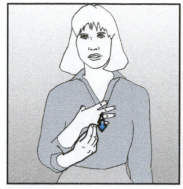

WHITE

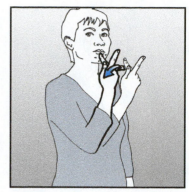

PINK

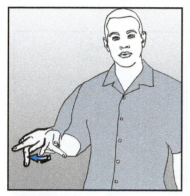

PURPLE

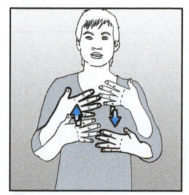

GRAY

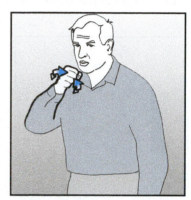

ORANGE

▶ **Clothing**

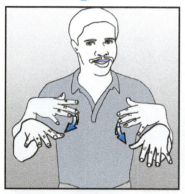

DRESS, clothes

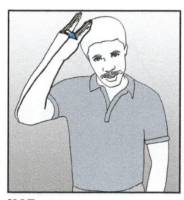

HAT, cap

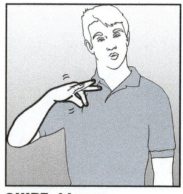

SHIRT, blouse

▶ **Physical Features and Attributes**

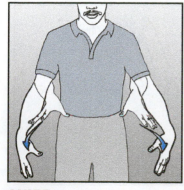

SKIRT

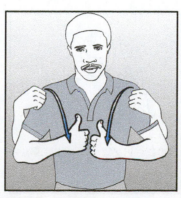

COAT, jacket

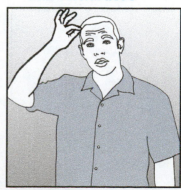

HAIR

4

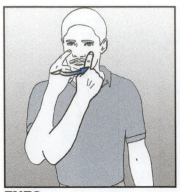

EYES

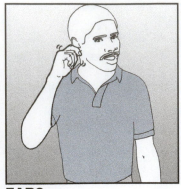

EARS

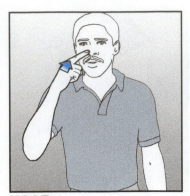

NOSE

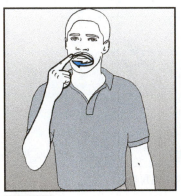

MOUTH

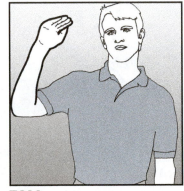

TALL

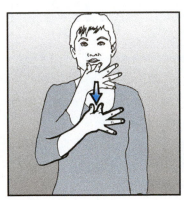

THIN

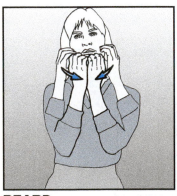

BEARD

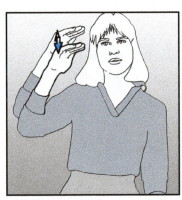

SMALL, short

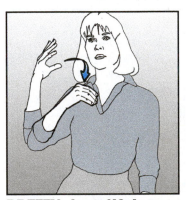

PRETTY, beautiful

▶ **Personality Attributes**

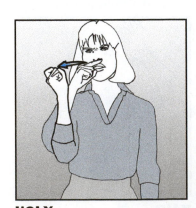

UGLY

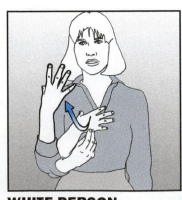

WHITE-PERSON

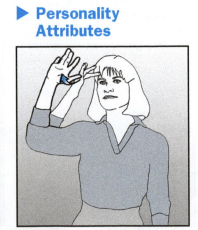

SMART, intelligent

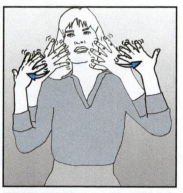

FRIENDLY, pleasant, cheerful

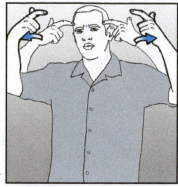

ARROGANT, egotistical

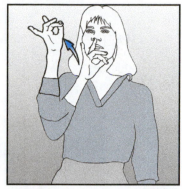

STUCK-UP, snob, snobbish

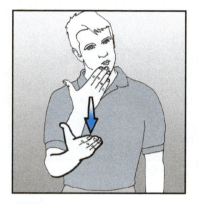

GOOD

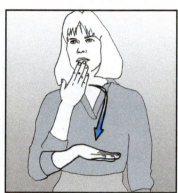

BAD, evil

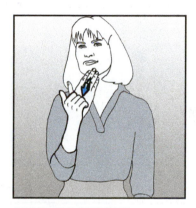

SWEET-NATURED

▶ **Other Vocabulary**

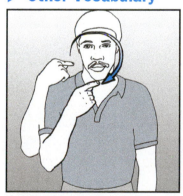

APPEARANCE, looks, face

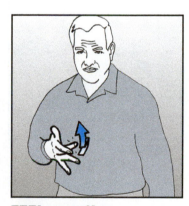

FEEL, emotion

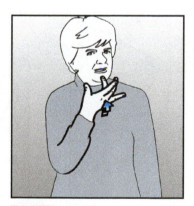

TASTE, prefer

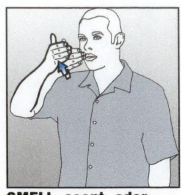

SMELL, scent, odor

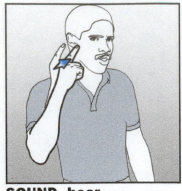

SOUND, hear

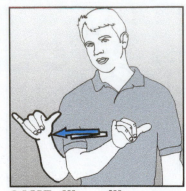

SAME, like, alike

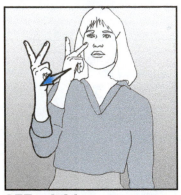

SEE, sight

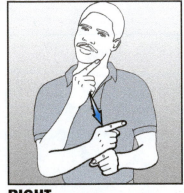

RIGHT

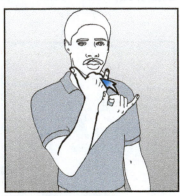

WRONG, mistake

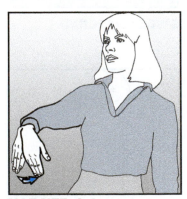

NOT-YET, late

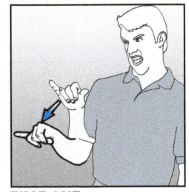

THAT-ONE

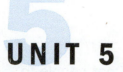

UNIT 5

Requests

In this unit, you make different kinds of requests. First, you will learn how to make polite commands.

You will learn about verb pairs and noun–verb pairs.

And you will learn how to use DON'T-MIND and FOR ME in making requests.

In a culture note, you will read how Deaf people get the attention of others.

5

POLITE COMMANDS

(Several people are in a room.)

Alex: YOU, PLEASE FLASH-LIGHTS.

(Lisa flashes the lights on and off.)

Alex: YOU, CLOSE-DOOR. FEEL A-LITTLE COLD.

(Lisa closes the door.)

Alex: THANK-YOU. PLEASE SIT.

(Everyone sits down.)

Alex: NOW GO-AHEAD START.

Key Structures

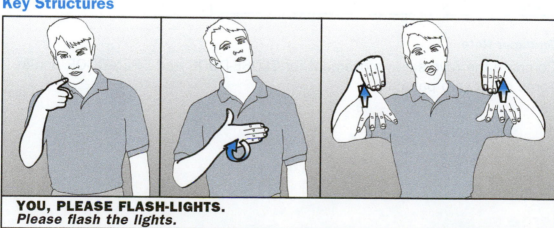

YOU, PLEASE FLASH-LIGHTS.
Please flash the lights.

Culture Note

Flashing the lights on and off in a room is a common way for Deaf people to get each other's attention. This is usually done within groups, but can be done to get the attention of someone alone in a room.

However, a preferred way of getting the attention of someone is a small wave of the hand in the person's field of vision. Waving both hands at once can also get the attention of a group if flashing the lights isn't possible.

At home Deaf people get each other's attention primarily by waving the hand or sharply rapping on a surface such as a table with the fist or flat of the hand so that the other person can feel it. Sometimes a well-measured stomp of a foot on the floor is acceptable.

Another way to get someone's attention is to touch or tap lightly on the arm, shoulder, or knee.

A note of caution: waving, rapping, and stomping are usually used in ways which do not disturb people who hear in public places and can be quite annoying even to Deaf people if overdone.

Clapping the hands to get someone's attention is neither effective nor socially acceptable.

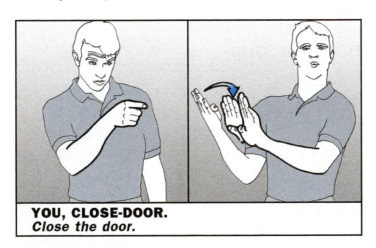

YOU, CLOSE-DOOR.
Close the door.

Grammar Note

Compare the reversal in movement for CLOSE-DOOR and OPEN-DOOR and in some other verb pairs:

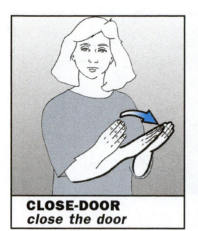

CLOSE-DOOR
close the door

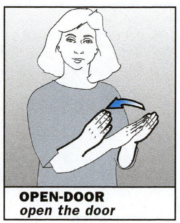

OPEN-DOOR
open the door

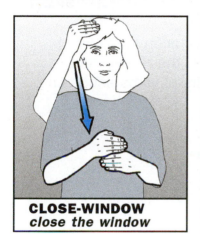

CLOSE-WINDOW
close the window

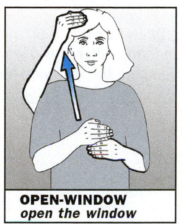

OPEN-WINDOW
open the window

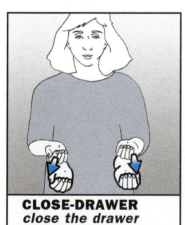

CLOSE-DRAWER
close the drawer

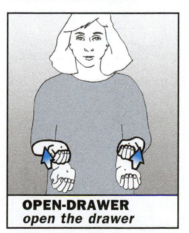

OPEN-DRAWER
open the drawer

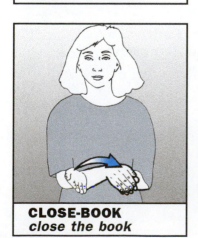

CLOSE-BOOK
close the book

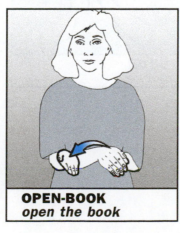

OPEN-BOOK
open the book

5

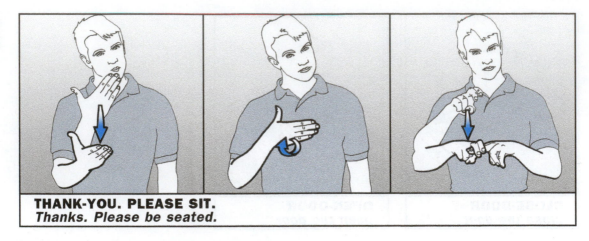

THANK-YOU. PLEASE SIT.
Thanks. Please be seated.

Grammar Note

Some verbs such as CLOSE/OPEN-DOOR and SIT have noun forms which differ in movement. The noun forms differ in two ways: their movement is repeated and it is smaller. Compare the following pairs of verbs and nouns:

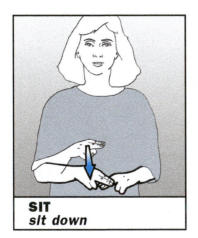

SIT
sit down

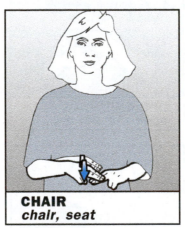

CHAIR
chair, seat

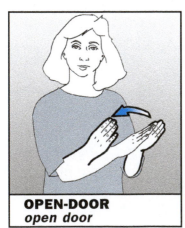

OPEN-DOOR
open door

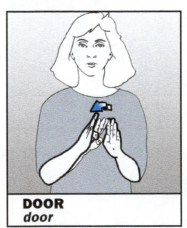

DOOR
door

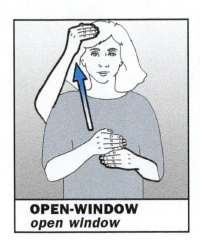

OPEN-WINDOW
open window

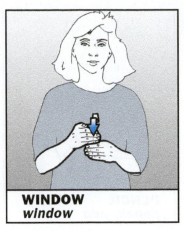

WINDOW
window

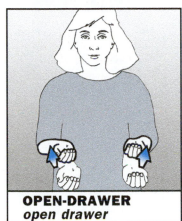

OPEN-DRAWER
open drawer

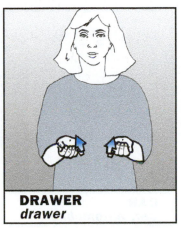

DRAWER
drawer

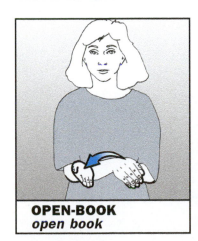

OPEN-BOOK
open book

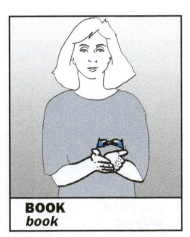

BOOK
book

Some verbs have repeated movement. As in the above, the noun forms have repeated and smaller movements. Compare the following pairs of verbs and nouns:

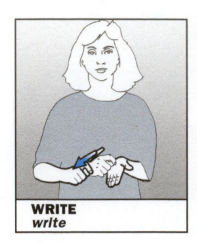

WRITE
write

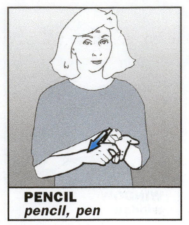

PENCIL
pencil, pen

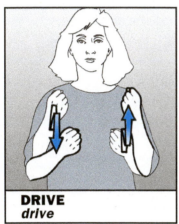

DRIVE
drive

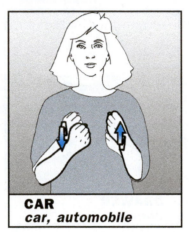

CAR
car, automobile

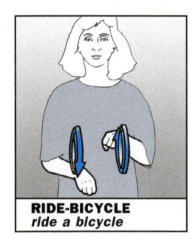

RIDE-BICYCLE
ride a bicycle

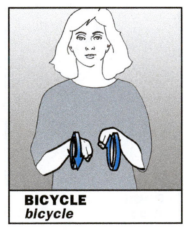

BICYCLE
bicycle

Exercise 5A

a. Working in pairs, tell your partner to do the following things:

1. open a window
2. stand up
3. sit down
4. spell his/her name
5. close a window
6. close a door
7. bring you a chair
8. show you his/her pencil

b. Following the prompt, make comments about each of the following:

Prompt: book, open

_____t_____
BOOK THERE, OPEN-BOOK.

1. window, close
2. door, open
3. drawer, open
4. chair, bring here, sit
5. window, open
6. book, close
7. drawer, close
8. bicycle, ride
9. pencil, write
10. car, drive

REQUESTS TO DO SOMETHING

_____q_____
Lisa: DON'T-MIND IT OPEN-WINDOW?

Chris: SURE!

_____q_____
Lisa: THANK-YOU. DON'T-MIND 1-MORE?

          whq
Chris: WHAT?

_____q_____
Lisa: GARBAGE THROW-OUT, CAN YOU?

Chris: O-K, YOU-OWE-ME YOU.

Key Structures

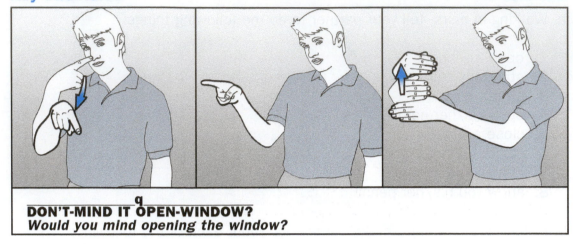

                   q
DON'T-MIND IT OPEN-WINDOW?
Would you mind opening the window?

Note

DON'T-MIND is used in the above example as a polite way to make a request for someone else to do something. DON'T-MIND is also used to ask if it's all right for you to do something as in:

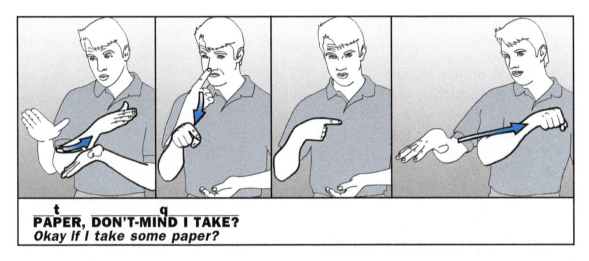

  t   q
PAPER, DON'T-MIND I TAKE?
Okay if I take some paper?

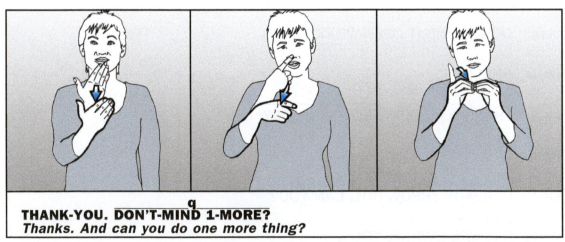

                   q
THANK-YOU. DON'T-MIND 1-MORE?
Thanks. And can you do one more thing?

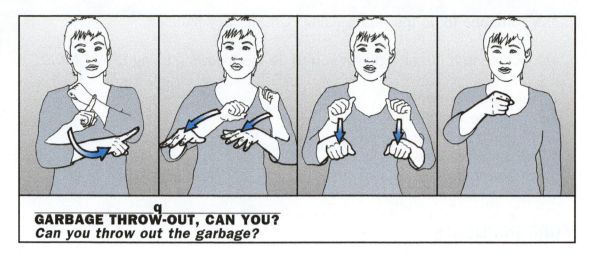

q
GARBAGE THROW-OUT, CAN YOU?
Can you throw out the garbage?

Note

Another way of asking someone to do something is to use FOR ME as in the sentence below:

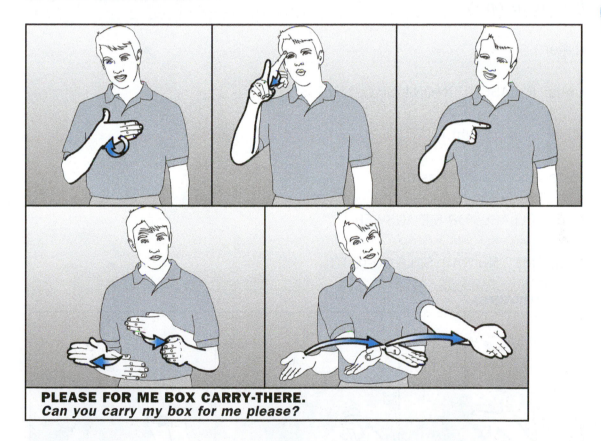

PLEASE FOR ME BOX CARRY-THERE.
Can you carry my box for me please?

Exercise 5B

q
a. Ask someone to do the following using DON'T-MIND:

1. move a chair
2. give you your coat
3. open the door

b. Ask someone to do the above using FOR ME. Say please.

c. Ask someone if it's all right for you to do the following using DON'T-MIND.

1. take his/her pencil
2. close the window
3. throw away a bag
4. take his/her chair
5. close the door

MORE REQUESTS

Chris: PLEASE TURN-ON T-V.

(Lisa turns on TV.)

(Later.)

Chris: PLEASE TURN-ON-LIGHT. CAN'T SEE.

(Lisa turns on light.)

(Later phone lights flash.)

Chris: PLEASE FOR ME ANSWER.

    _q_
Lisa: ME? NO-WAY. SELF GO-TO-IT!

Key Structures

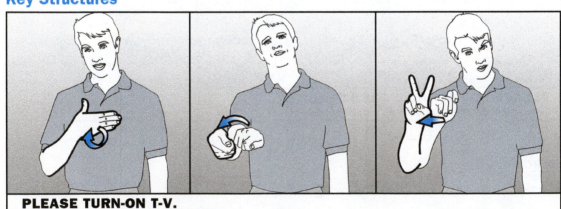

PLEASE TURN-ON T-V.
Please turn on the television.

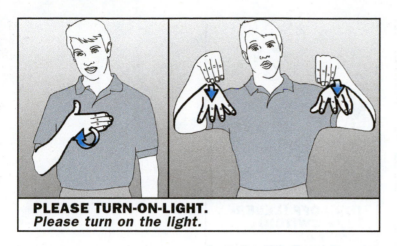

PLEASE TURN-ON-LIGHT.
Please turn on the light.

Note

As with OPEN-DOOR and CLOSE-DOOR, some other verbs involving turning something on and off use a reversal of the movement. Compare the following:

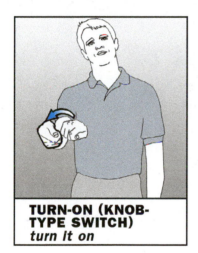

TURN-ON (KNOB-TYPE SWITCH)
turn it on

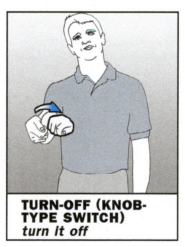

TURN-OFF (KNOB-TYPE SWITCH)
turn it off

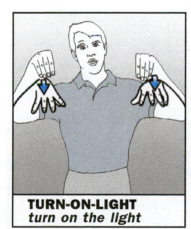

TURN-ON-LIGHT
turn on the light

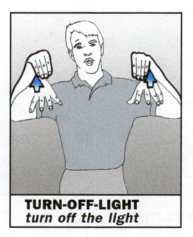

TURN-OFF-LIGHT
turn off the light

5

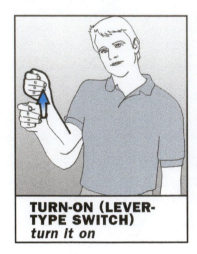

TURN-ON (LEVER-TYPE SWITCH)
turn it on

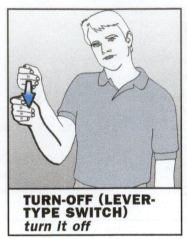

TURN-OFF (LEVER-TYPE SWITCH)
turn it off

However, the movement for turning on or off a push-button type switch is the same:

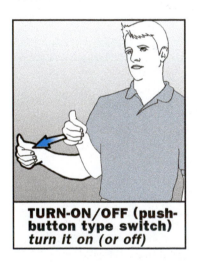

TURN-ON/OFF (push-button type switch)
turn it on (or off)

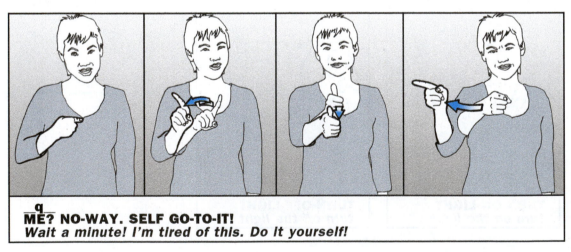

q
ME? NO-WAY. SELF GO-TO-IT!
Wait a minute! I'm tired of this. Do it yourself!

Exercise 5C

a. Working in pairs, ask your partner to turn on the following:

1. a television with a knob-type switch
2. a television with a push-button type switch
3. a light on the ceiling
4. a table-lamp type light
5. a light switch of the lever type

b. Then ask your partner to turn off each of the above. Your partner should tell you to turn each item off yourself as in the prompt:

Prompt: SELF TURN-OFF-_____.

VOCABULARY

▶ Verb Pairs

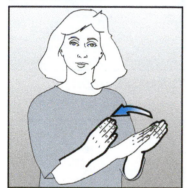

OPEN-DOOR

CLOSE-DOOR

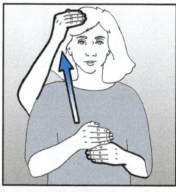

OPEN-WINDOW

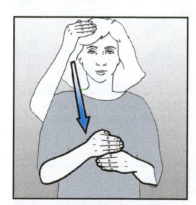

CLOSE-WINDOW

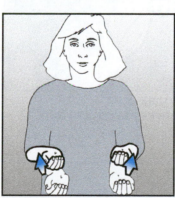

OPEN-DRAWER

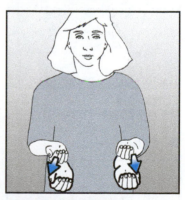

CLOSE-DRAWER

5

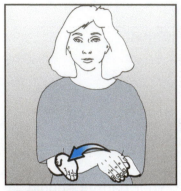
OPEN-BOOK

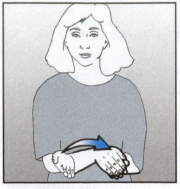
CLOSE-BOOK

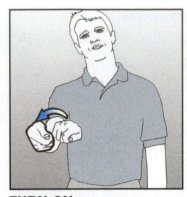
TURN-ON
(knob-type switch)

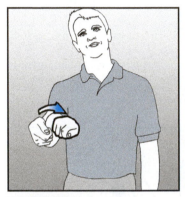
TURN-OFF
(knob-type switch)

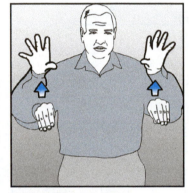
TURN-ON (light)

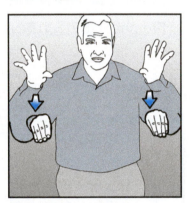
TURN-OFF (light)

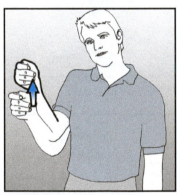
TURN-ON
(lever-type switch)

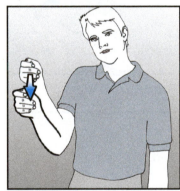
TURN-OFF
(lever-type switch)

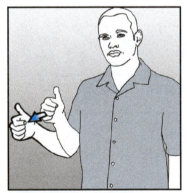
TURN-ON/OFF (push-
button type switch)

▶ **Other Verbs**

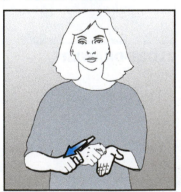
WRITE

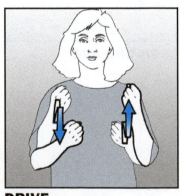
DRIVE

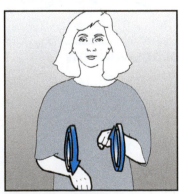
RIDE-BICYCLE

▶ Nouns

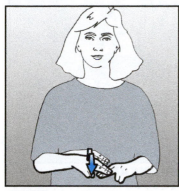

CHAIR

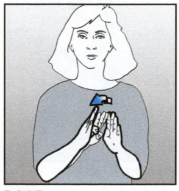

DOOR

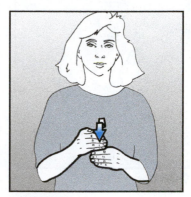

WINDOW

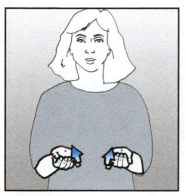

DRAWER

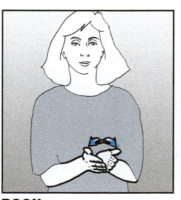

BOOK

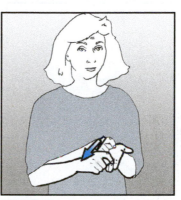

PENCIL, pen

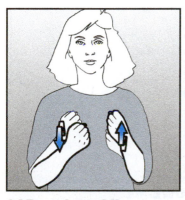

CAR, automobile

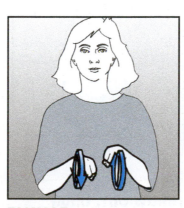

BICYCLE

▶ Other Vocabulary

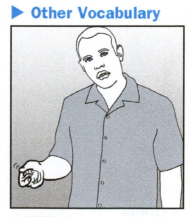

A-LITTLE

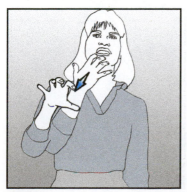

HOT

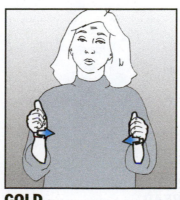

COLD

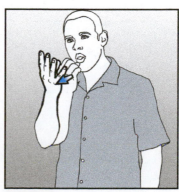

WARM

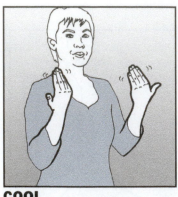

COOL

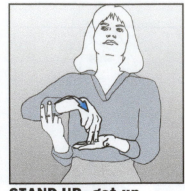

STAND-UP, get up

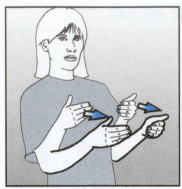

GO-AHEAD, go on, proceed

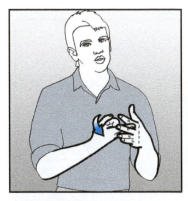

START, begin, initiate, originate

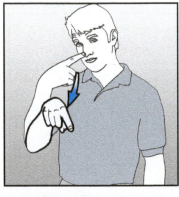

DON'T-MIND, don't care

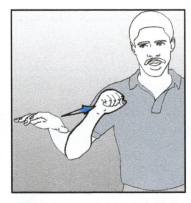

TAKE

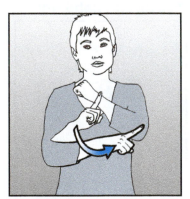

GARBAGE

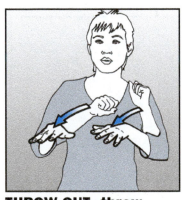

THROW-OUT, throw away

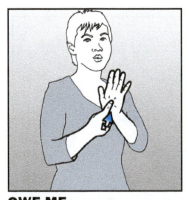

OWE-ME

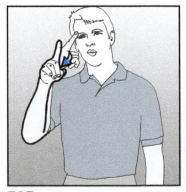

FOR

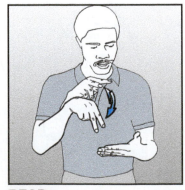

READ

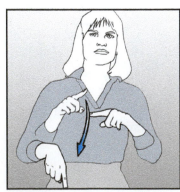

CAN'T

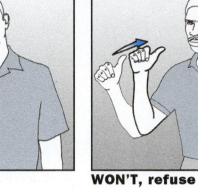

ANSWER, respond

SELF

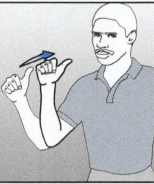

WON'T, refuse

5

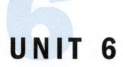

UNIT 6

Expressing Yourself

In this unit, you will learn various ways to express your feelings, opinions, and preferences.

You will use ALL-DAY and ALL-NIGHT forms.

You will learn about negative incorporation such as DON'T-KNOW.

You will also learn about the use of modals and their position in sentences.

HOW YOU FEEL

Pat: GOOD-MORNING! HOW YOU?
                    _____q_____

Alex: I SO-SO. YOU?
             __q__

Pat: I FINE. WRONG?
             __whq__

Alex: ALL-NIGHT I ROLL-AROUND. I TIRED I.

Pat: OH-I-SEE. SYMPATHIZE-WITH. WANT COFFEE?
                         _____q_____

Alex: YES!

Key Structures

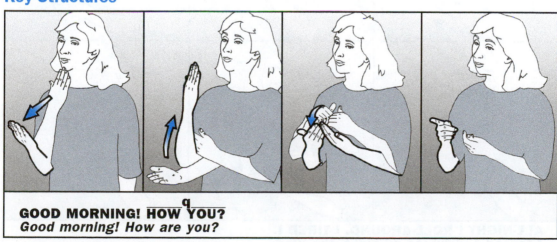

GOOD MORNING! HOW YOU?
Good morning! How are you?

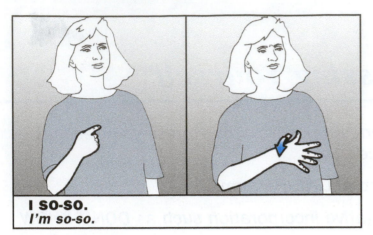

I SO-SO.
I'm so-so.

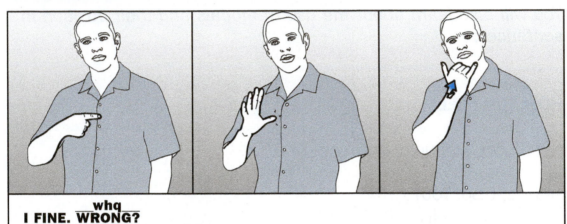

I FINE. $\overline{\text{whq}}$ **WRONG?**
I'm fine. What's wrong?

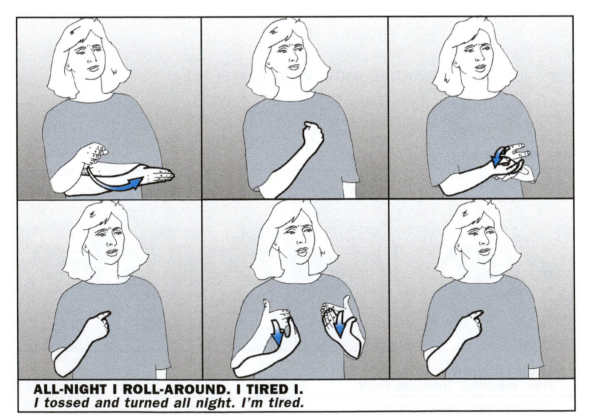

ALL-NIGHT I ROLL-AROUND. I TIRED I.
I tossed and turned all night. I'm tired.

Note

The sweeping movement used to indicate "all night" or "overnight" in ALL-NIGHT is also used with DAY, MORNING, AFTERNOON, and EVENING. Compare the following:

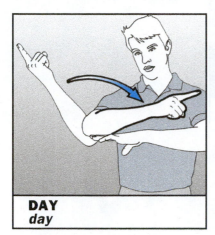

DAY
day

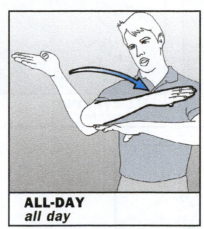

ALL-DAY
all day

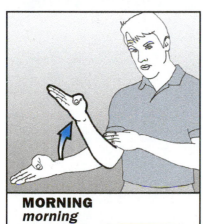

MORNING
morning

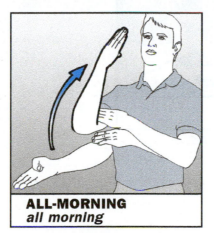

ALL-MORNING
all morning

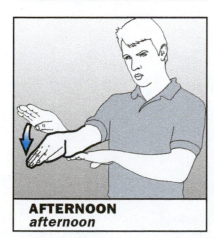

AFTERNOON
afternoon

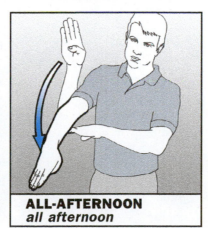

ALL-AFTERNOON
all afternoon

6

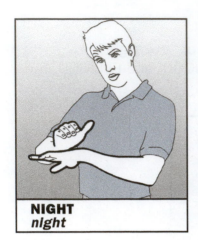

NIGHT
night

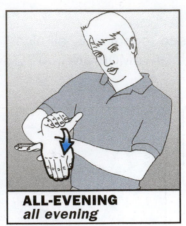

ALL-EVENING
all evening

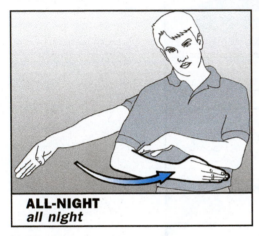

ALL-NIGHT
all night

Exercise 6A

In response to "How are you?," say that you are:

1. sleepy
2. tired
3. hungry
4. fine
5. feeling good
6. cold
7. hot
8. so-so
9. cranky
10. sick

OPINIONS AND PREFERENCES

Lisa: WOW. APPEARANCE MAD YOU. $\overline{\text{WRONG}}^{\text{whq}}$?

Pat: J-O-H-N NOT SHOW-UP.

Lisa: OH-I-SEE. $\overline{\text{HE LATE}}^{q}$?

Pat: YES. NOT LIKE I.

Lisa: NOT SURPRISED I.

Key Structures

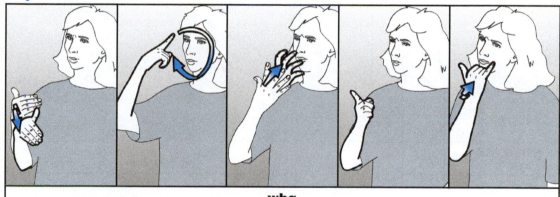

WOW. APPEARANCE MAD YOU. $\overline{\text{WRONG}}^{\text{whq}}$?
Wow. You look mad. What's wrong?

Note

WOW is used to indicate the degree of impact or reaction a person feels upon experiencing something. It is not limited to a reaction of delight. For example:

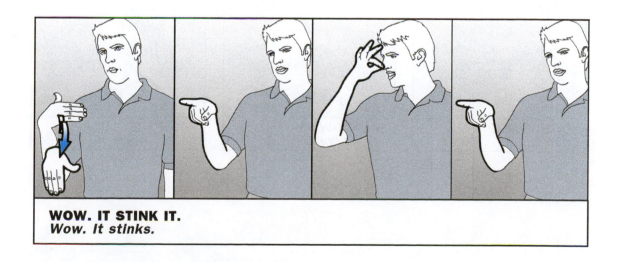

WOW. IT STINK IT.
Wow. It stinks.

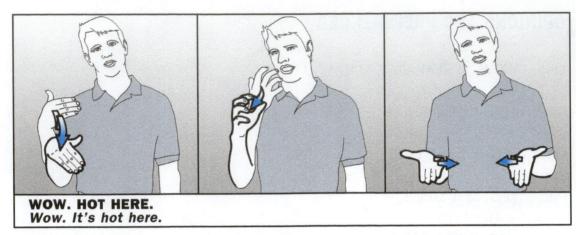

WOW. HOT HERE.
Wow. It's hot here.

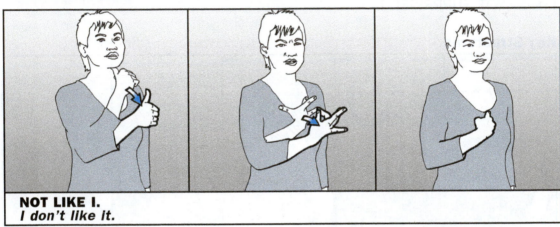

NOT LIKE I.
I don't like it.

Grammar Note

The negatives of LIKE, WANT, and KNOW can be made with a twisting movement outward from the body, as in the following:

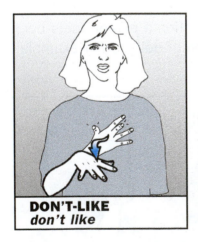

DON'T-LIKE
don't like

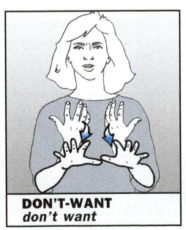

DON'T-WANT
don't want

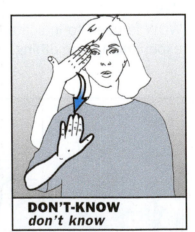

DON'T-KNOW
don't know

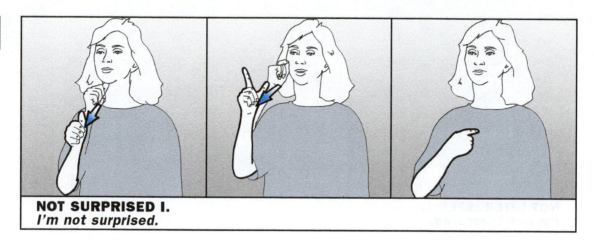

NOT SURPRISED I.
I'm not surprised.

Grammar Note

The above structure is often used to express negative feelings or respond to inquiries about feelings. Some other examples are:

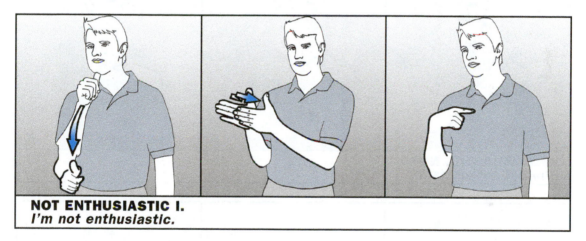

NOT ENTHUSIASTIC I.
I'm not enthusiastic.

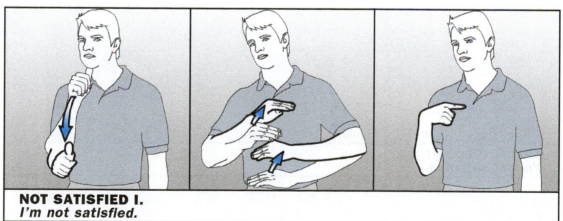

NOT SATISFIED I.
I'm not satisfied.

6

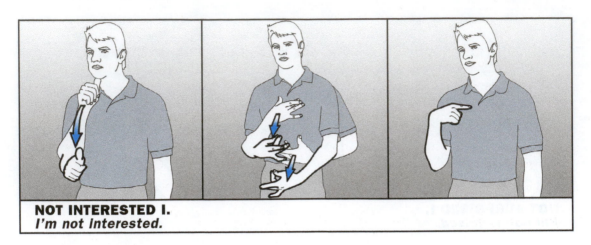

NOT INTERESTED I.
I'm not interested.

Or, NOT can come after the adjective as in:

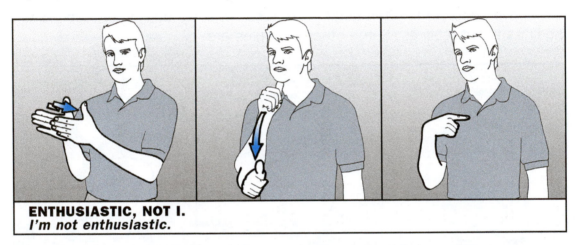

ENTHUSIASTIC, NOT I.
I'm not enthusiastic.

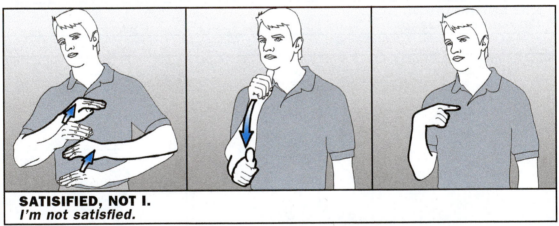

SATISIFIED, NOT I.
I'm not satisfied.

Exercise 6B

a. Working in pairs, express the following feelings to your partner:

1. satisfaction
2. happiness
3. anger
4. sadness
5. surprise
6. interest

b. Still working in pairs, tell your partner that you are not:

1. happy
2. satisfied
3. surprised
4. enthusiastic
5. excited
6. interested

ANXIETY

Lisa: I NERVOUS I.

Chris: STOP WORRY!

Lisa: PASS TEST MUST I.

Chris: PASS WILL YOU. CALM-DOWN.

Lisa: FLUNK WILL I.

Key Structures

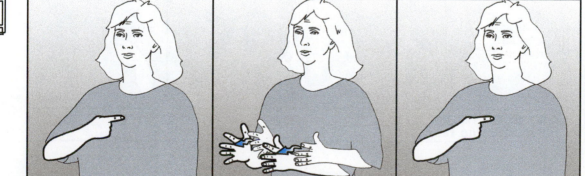

I NERVOUS I.
I'm nervous.

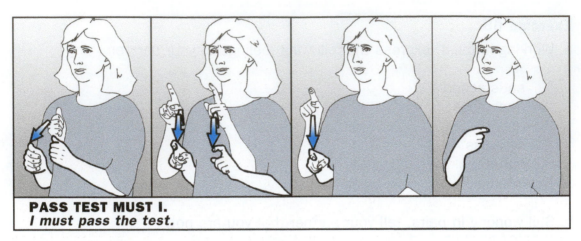

PASS TEST MUST I.
I must pass the test.

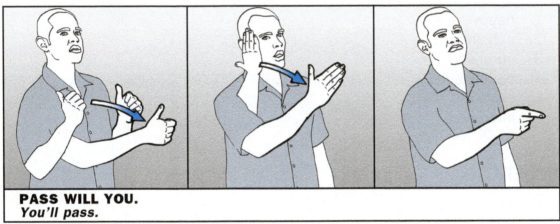

PASS WILL YOU.
You'll pass.

Grammar Note

Modals such as MUST, SHOULD, CAN, and WILL can be used in the following ways:

1. Before the verb:

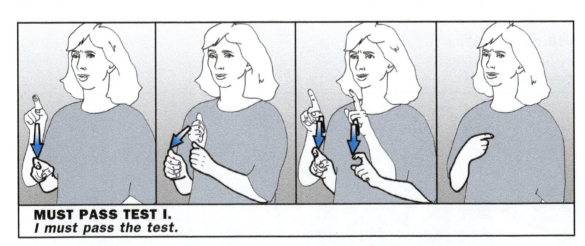

MUST PASS TEST I.
I must pass the test.

2. After the verb:

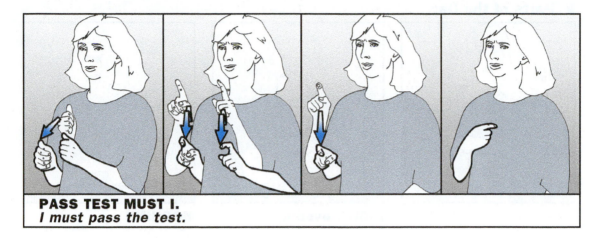

PASS TEST MUST I.
I must pass the test.

3. Before the verb and repeated at the end of the sentence:

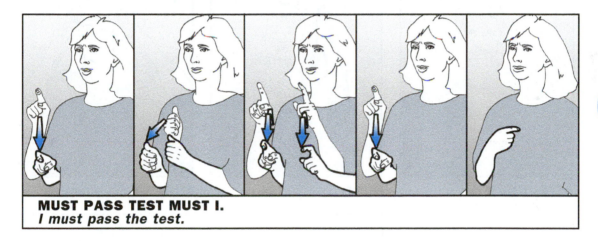

MUST PASS TEST MUST I.
I must pass the test.

Exercise 6C

Following the prompt, make as many sentences using MUST, WILL, CAN, or SHOULD as you can:

Prompt: TAKE-UP TEST WILL I.

1. sleep all day
2. help the teacher
3. calm down
4. take test
5. show up
6. go to class

VOCABULARY

▶ **Parts of the Day**

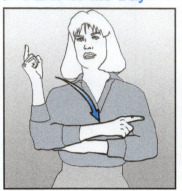

DAY

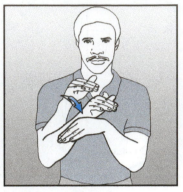

NIGHT, evening

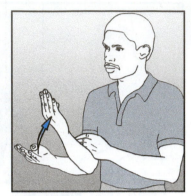

MORNING

▶ **Adjectives**

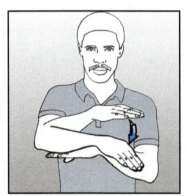

AFTERNOON

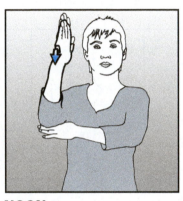

NOON

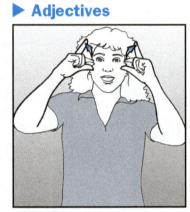

SURPRISED, amazed

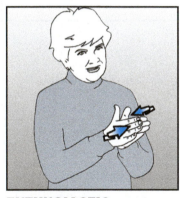

ENTHUSIASTIC, eager, motivated

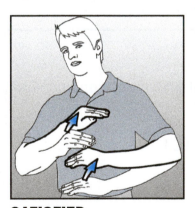

SATISFIED

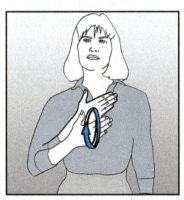

HAPPY

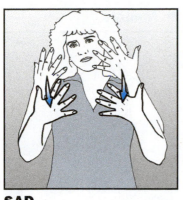

SAD

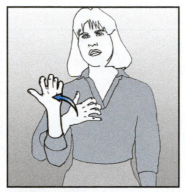

MAD, angry

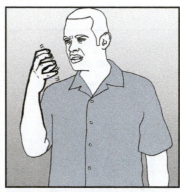

CRANKY, mad, grouchy

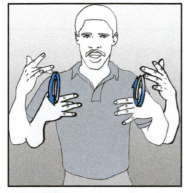

EXCITED

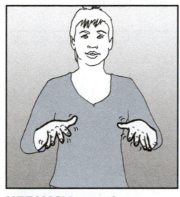

NERVOUS, anxious

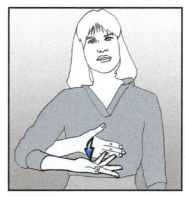

UPSET

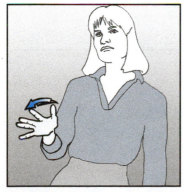

SO-SO

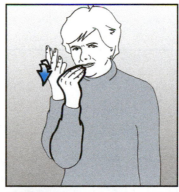

SLEEPY

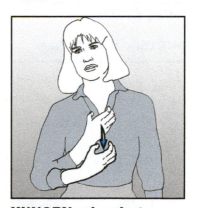

HUNGRY, starving

▶ **Negatives**

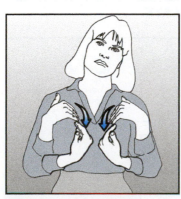

TIRED, exhausted

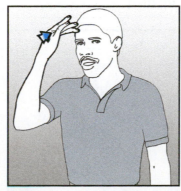

SICK

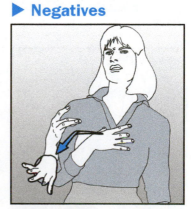

DON'T-LIKE

6

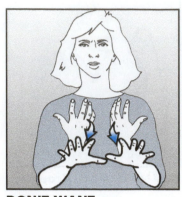

DON'T-WANT

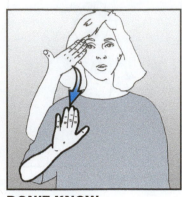

DON'T-KNOW

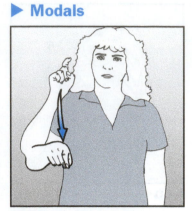

MUST, have to

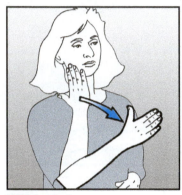

WILL, future

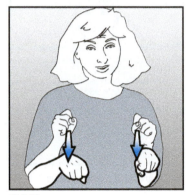

CAN

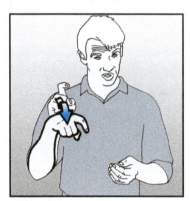

SHOULD

▶ **Other Vocabulary**

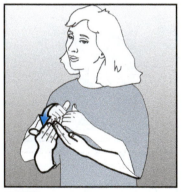

HOW

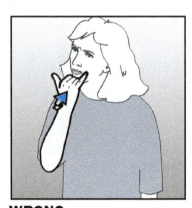

WRONG

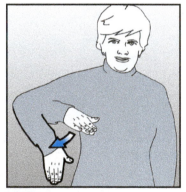

LATE

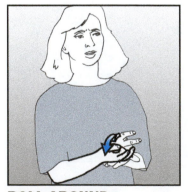

ROLL-AROUND

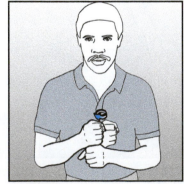

COFFEE

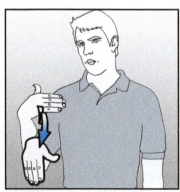

WOW

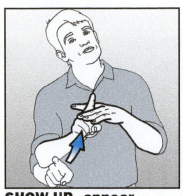

SHOW-UP, appear

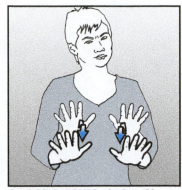

CALM-DOWN, take it easy

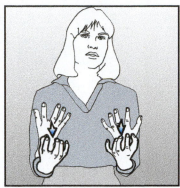

WANT, DESIRE

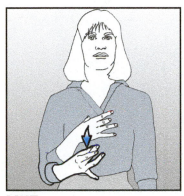

LIKE

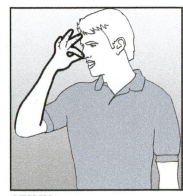

STINK

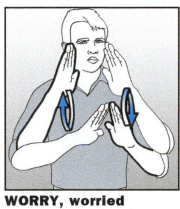

WORRY, worried

6

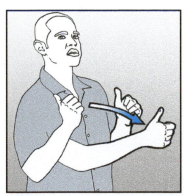

PASS

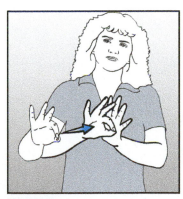

FLUNK

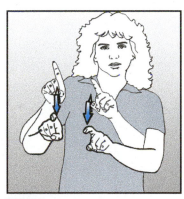

TEST, exam

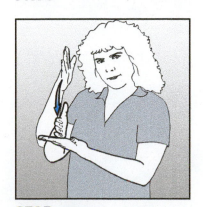

STOP, cease

UNIT 7

More Descriptions

In this unit, you will learn about classifiers that show the size and shape of an object and classifiers that indicate how an object is moved or placed.

You will also use classifiers that indicate the location of objects in relation to each other.

And you will learn how to show quantity by using numbers or quantifiers such as MANY, SOME, SEVERAL, or A-FEW.

OBJECTS AND THEIR LOCATION

Chris: MY GLASS I CL:C>-PUT-THERE. GONE.

Lisa: I CL:C>-CARRY-TO KITCHEN.

_____whq_____
Chris: CL:C>-THERE WHERE?

Lisa: TABLE THERE, CL:C>-THERE.

Key Structures

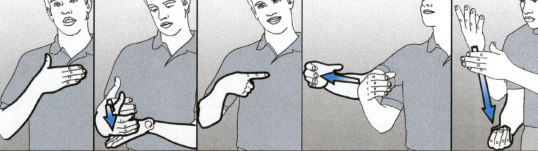

MY GLASS I CL:C>-PUT-THERE. GONE.
I put my glass there. Now it's gone.

Grammar Note

Some predicates have classifiers that show the size and shape of an object. For example, in the sentence above, the classifier, CL:C>, represents a cylinder-like shape the size of a glass, cup, or bottle. Compare the properties of some classifier predicates:

83

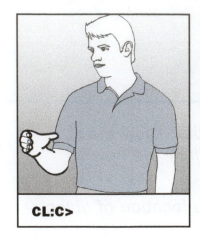

CL:C>

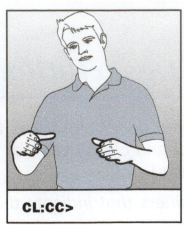

CL:CC>

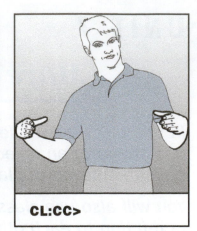

CL:CC>

Cylinder-like shape such as a glass, cup, bottle, large candle.

Large cylinder-like shape such as a lamppost, coffee can, or flower pot.

Larger cylinder-like shape such as a bucket, trash can, or drum.

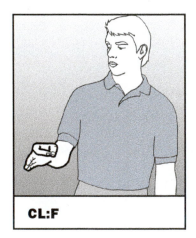

CL:F

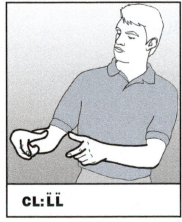

CL:ÏL

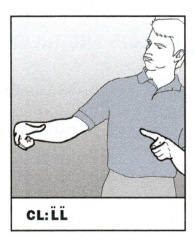

CL:ÏL

Small round, flat disk-like shape such as a coin or button.

Round, flat disk-like shape such as a saucer, clockface, or circular picture.

Large round, flat disk-like shape such as a larger platter, place mat, or frame.

Note that the predicate also indicates the location of the object as in CL:C>-PUT-THERE in the sentence on page 83.

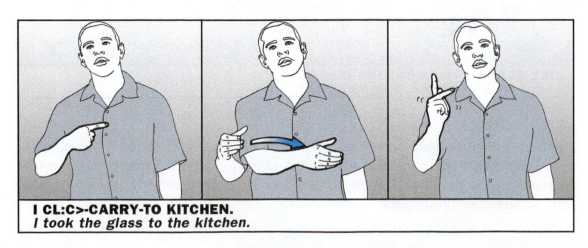

I CL:C>-CARRY-TO KITCHEN.
I took the glass to the kitchen.

Grammar Note

Some predicates with instrument classifiers indicate how an object is moved or placed as in CL:C>-CARRY-TO in the previous example. Some other such classifiers are:

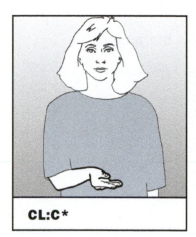

CL:C*

For objects such as a book, a flat box, a box of candy, or a stack of paper.

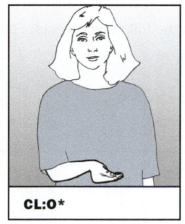

CL:O*

For thin, flat objects such as a sheet of paper or a thin magazine.

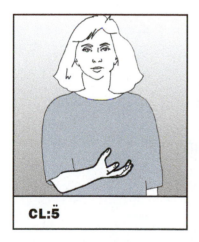

CL:5̈

For small round objects such as a baseball, an apple, or an orange.

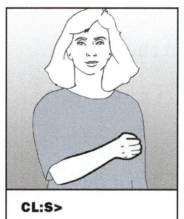

CL:S>

For handle-like objects or objects with handles such as a broom, a pitcher, or a mug.

Exercise 7A

a. Working in pairs, indicate the size and location of the following objects. Follow the prompt.

Prompt: a glass

CL:C>-THERE.

1. a can of soda
2. a silver dollar
3. a wastebasket
4. a large pizza
5. a thick candle

b. Indicate that you moved the following objects. Follow the prompt.

Prompt: a glass

CL:C*-CARRY-TO.

1. a book
2. a thick stack of paper
3. a cup
4. a peach
5. a pitcher
6. a box of candy
7. a mug
8. a newspaper
9. a letter
10. an orange

OBJECTS, NUMBER, AND LOCATION

                           t

Chris: APPLE CL:5̈-NEXT-TO-CL-5̈-THERE, NOT TOUCH YOU.

Lisa: BETTER YOU CL:5̈-NEXT-TO-CL-5̈-PUT-THERE HIDE.

Chris: NO. I LEAVE-THERE. YOU NOT TOUCH.

Key Structures

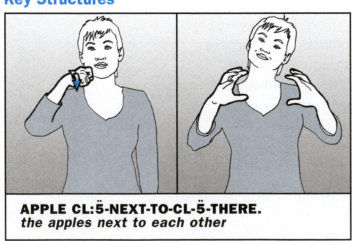

APPLE CL:5̈-NEXT-TO-CL-5̈-THERE.
the apples next to each other

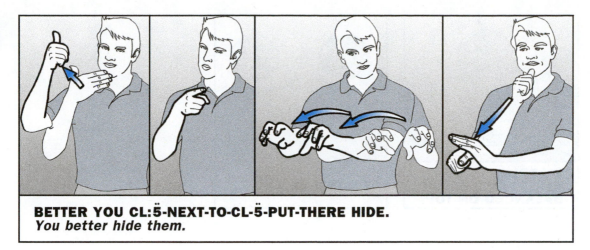

BETTER YOU CL:5̈-NEXT-TO-CL:5̈-PUT-THERE HIDE.
You better hide them.

Grammar Note

Classifier predicates can be used to indicate the location of objects in relation to each other as in CL-5̈-NEXT-TO-CL:5̈-PUT-THERE above. The sentence below shows the relationship of more than two objects:

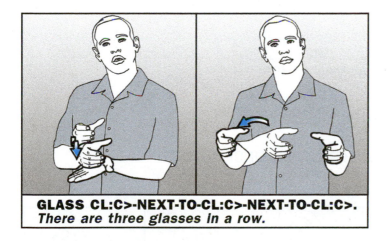

GLASS CL:C>-NEXT-TO-CL:C>-NEXT-TO-CL:C>.
There are three glasses in a row.

Exercise 7B

Describe the location of the objects in the following pictures:

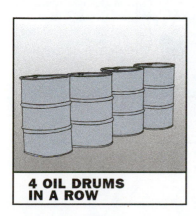

4 OIL DRUMS IN A ROW

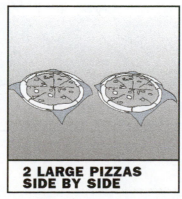

2 LARGE PIZZAS SIDE BY SIDE

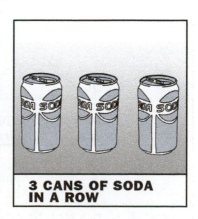

3 CANS OF SODA IN A ROW

7

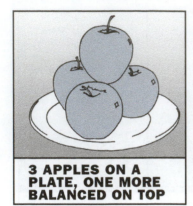

3 APPLES ON A PLATE, ONE MORE BALANCED ON TOP

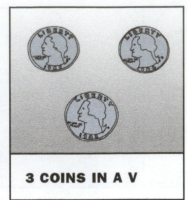

3 COINS IN A V

HOW MANY

_____q_____
Lisa: CLOTHES YOU HAVE? I WASH-CLOTHES.

Chris: YES. HAVE SOME. I BRING-HERE.

(Chris brings a pile of clothes.)

_____whq_____
Lisa: WOW! MANY SHIRT. HOW-MANY THERE?

Chris: I THINK 8. PLUS 4 PANTS.

Lisa: SEEM YOU NOT-YET WASH-CLOTHES SINCE 1-MONTH.

Key Structures

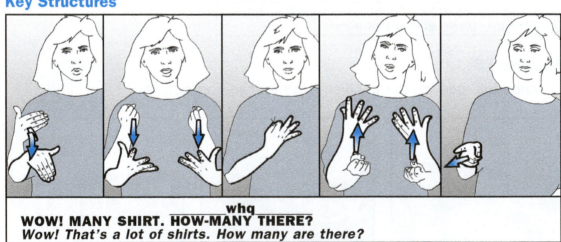

_____whq_____
WOW! MANY SHIRT. HOW-MANY THERE?
Wow! That's a lot of shirts. How many are there?

Grammar Note

One of the ways to show number (plural) is by using quantifiers such as MANY, SOME, SEVERAL, or A-FEW. These quantifiers can appear before or after the noun as in MANY SHIRT in the previous example or SHIRT MANY.

Note that the question form HOW-MANY? is made with the eyebrows squeezed together and the head tilted forward like other questions asking for information.

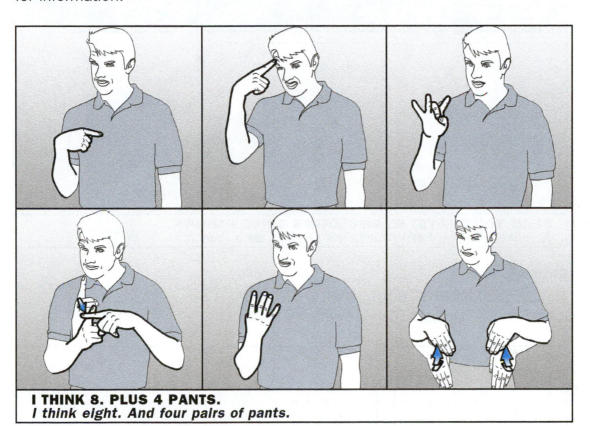

I THINK 8. PLUS 4 PANTS.
I think eight. And four pairs of pants.

Grammar Note

Another way to show number is by adding a number before or after the noun as in 4 PANTS above or PANTS 4.

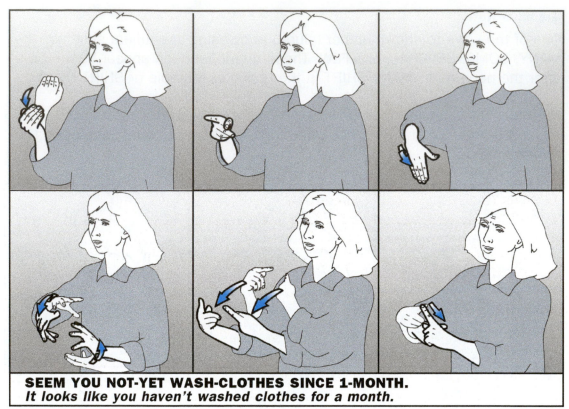

SEEM YOU NOT-YET WASH-CLOTHES SINCE 1-MONTH.
It looks like you haven't washed clothes for a month.

Grammar Note

The plural of MINUTE, HOUR, DAY, WEEK, MONTH can be made by incorporating numbers. Some examples are:

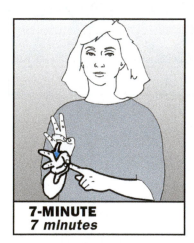

7-MINUTE
7 minutes

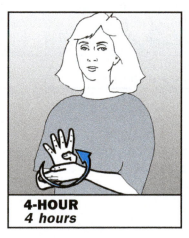

4-HOUR
4 hours

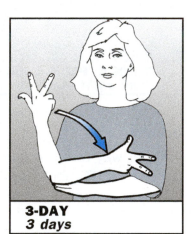

3-DAY
3 days

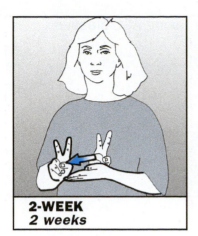

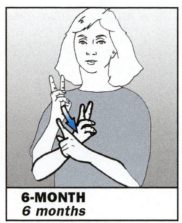

2-WEEK
2 weeks

6-MONTH
6 months

Only the numbers 1–9 can be incorporated in this way. But 10-MINUTE and similar incorporations, as in the following example, are acceptable usage in some places. For numbers greater than 9, use the number before the time sign as in:

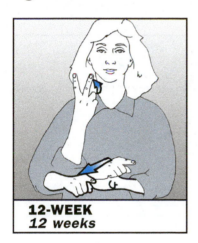

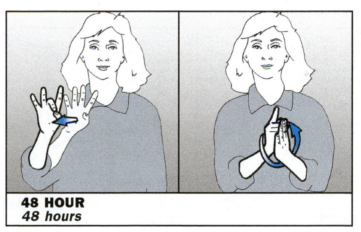

12-WEEK
12 weeks

48 HOUR
48 hours

Exercise 7C

a. Following the prompt, tell how many cars you have.

Prompt: four

HAVE FOUR CAR I.

1. many
2. several
3. three
4. two
5. a few
6. seven

b. Following the prompt, tell how long you have been taking ASL classes.

Prompt: 1 month

I TAKE-UP ASL SINCE 1-MONTH.

1. 2 weeks
2. 6 months
3. 11 weeks
4. 4 days
5. 24 hours
6. 2 hours
7. 3 minutes

VOCABULARY

▶ **Time**

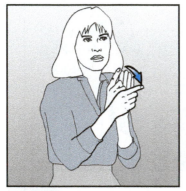

MINUTE

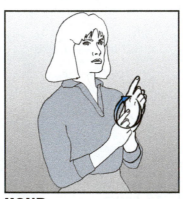

HOUR

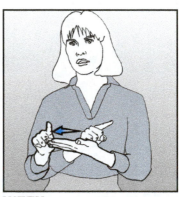

WEEK

▶ **Quantifiers**

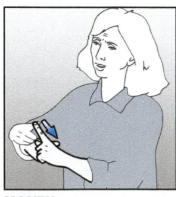

MONTH

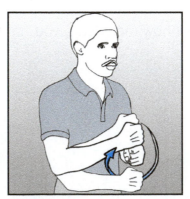

YEAR

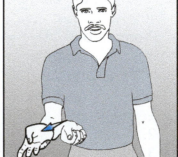

A-FEW

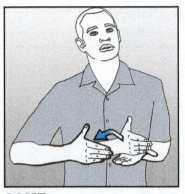
SOME

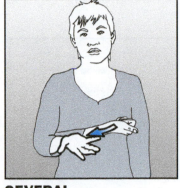
SEVERAL

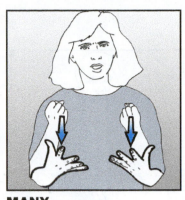
MANY

▶ **Fruit**

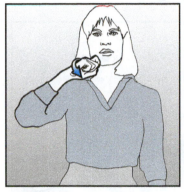
APPLE

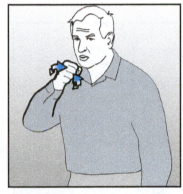
ORANGE

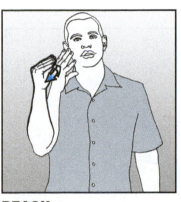
PEACH

▶ **Clothes**

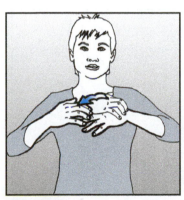
GRAPES

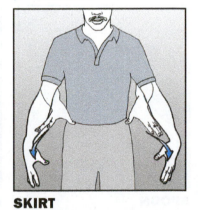
SKIRT

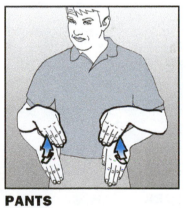
PANTS

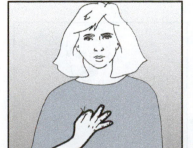
SHIRT

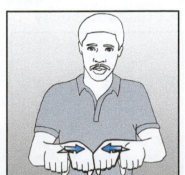
SHOES

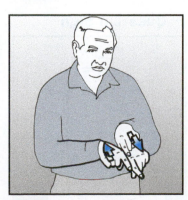
SOCK

7

▶ **Dishes and Silverware**

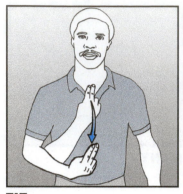

TIE

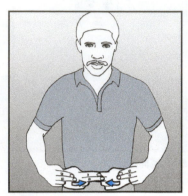

BELT

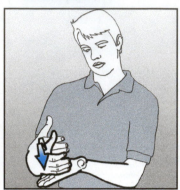

GLASS

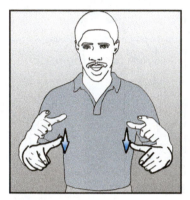

PLATE

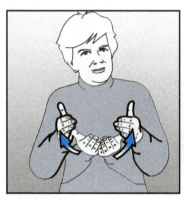

BOWL

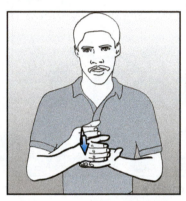

CUP

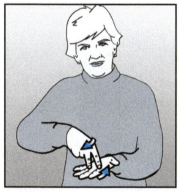

FORK

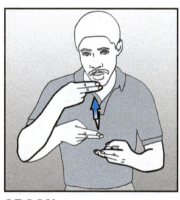

SPOON

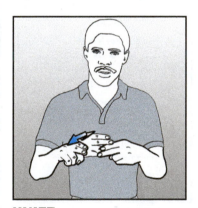

KNIFE

▶ **Question Sign**   ▶ **Other Vocabulary**

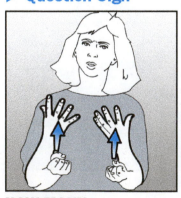

HOW-MANY

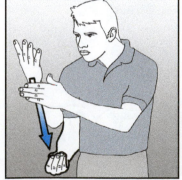

GONE

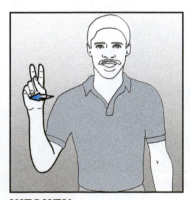

KITCHEN

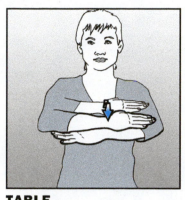

TABLE

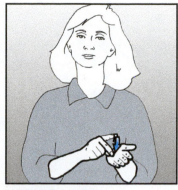

NEWSPAPER

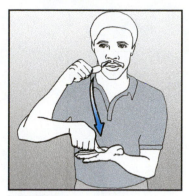

LETTER

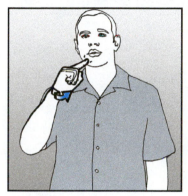

CANDY

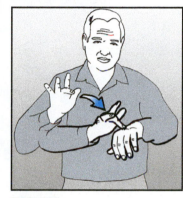

TOUCH

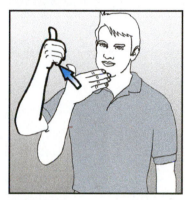

BETTER

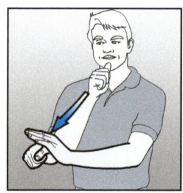

HIDE

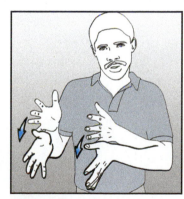

LEAVE-THERE, left

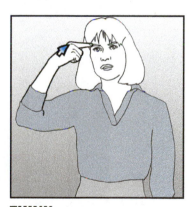

THINK

7

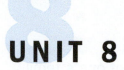

UNIT 8

Family and Friends

In this unit, you will ask for and give information about the family and family relationships. You will also talk about friends and acquaintances.

You will learn how to indicate past, present, and future tenses. You will learn how to use FINISH in several ways.

You will also learn about personal pronouns incorporating number, such as TWO-OF-YOU and THREE-OF-US.

In culture notes, you will learn about the common cultural practice of asking about hearing status and about establishing Deaf family ties.

FAMILY INFORMATION

Alex: $\overline{\text{MY FAMILY}}^{\;t}$ GATHER-TOGETHER TOMORROW. NOT-YET GATHER-TOGETHER SINCE TWO YEAR.

Chris: $\overline{\text{FAMILY DEAF?}}^{\;q}$

Alex: PARENTS DEAF. SISTER DEAF. TWO BROTHER, ONE DEAF, ONE HEARING.

Chris: $\overline{\text{BROTHER HEARING, SIGN?}}^{\;q}$

Alex: OF-COURSE!

Key Structures

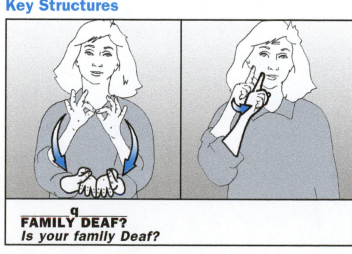

$\overline{\text{FAMILY DEAF?}}^{\;q}$
Is your family Deaf?

Culture Note

Asking for and giving information about whether the members of one's family are Deaf or hearing is a common cultural and social practice. Deaf people believe information such as this can contribute to understanding something about an individual and the individual's place among Deaf people.

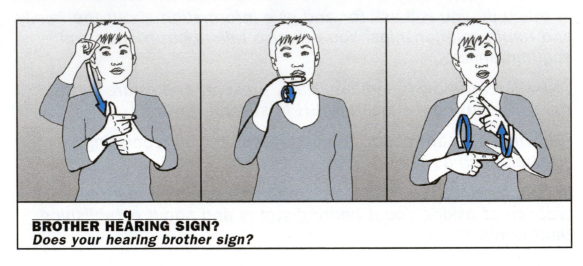

q
BROTHER HEARING SIGN?
Does your hearing brother sign?

Culture Note

Establishing whether hearing members of a Deaf person's family sign is part of finding out something about the Deaf person's experience. The conversation above has an interesting twist: Gloria's family is Deaf except for a hearing brother, so it is slightly ironic for Maria to ask if he can sign. Gloria's response of "Of course!" indicates the importance of sign to the family.

Exercise 8A

a. Working in pairs, ask your partner if her/his family members listed below are Deaf or hearing.

1. parents
2. mother
3. father
4. brother
5. sister
6. grandmother
7. grandfather
8. aunt
9. uncle
10. cousin

b. Ask your partner if each of the above can sign.

FAMILY RELATIONSHIPS

Alex: YESTERDAY I MEET-HIM YOUR HUSBAND. TWO-OF-YOU MARRY,

        _____whq_____
HOW-MANY YEAR?

Pat: TWO-OF-US MARRY 6 YEAR.

                                      _____q_____
Alex: WOW! I NOT REALIZE SINCE. HAVE CHILDREN?

Pat: TWO DAUGHTER, ONE SON.

        _____whq_____
Alex: DEAF, HEARING?

Pat: #ALL DEAF.

Key Structures

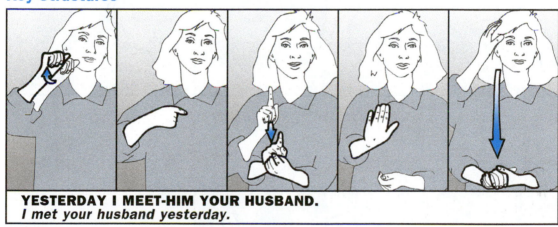

YESTERDAY I MEET-HIM YOUR HUSBAND.
I met your husband yesterday.

Grammar Note

One way to indicate past, present, or future tense is to use a tense sign at either the beginning or end of a sentence as in YESTERDAY I MEET-HIM YOUR HUSBAND above or I MEET-HIM YOUR HUSBAND YESTERDAY. Once the tense has been established in this way, it is not necessary to repeat a tense sign in each sentence. Some common tense signs from the vocabulary list are:

Present	Past	Future
NOW	YESTERDAY	TOMORROW
TODAY	BEFORE	WILL
	RECENT	LATER
	LONG-AGO	AFTER-A WHILE
		FAR-IN-FUTURE

8

Some examples are:

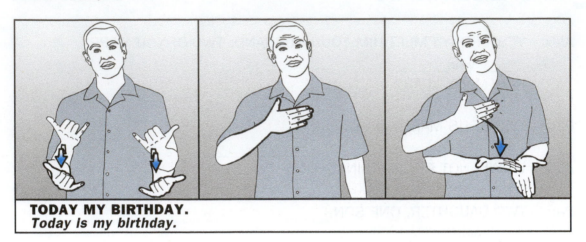

TODAY MY BIRTHDAY.
Today is my birthday.

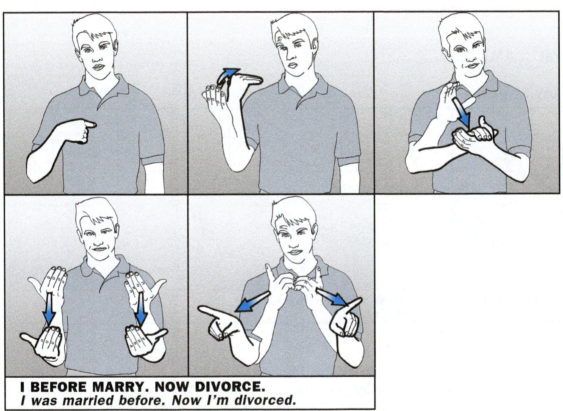

I BEFORE MARRY. NOW DIVORCE.
I was married before. Now I'm divorced.

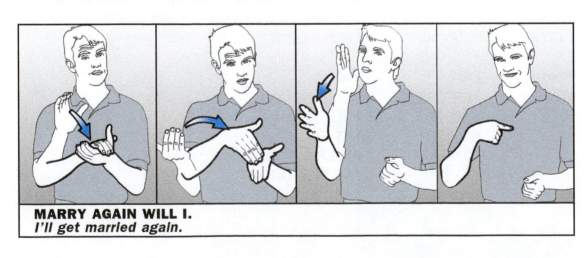

MARRY AGAIN WILL I.
I'll get married again.

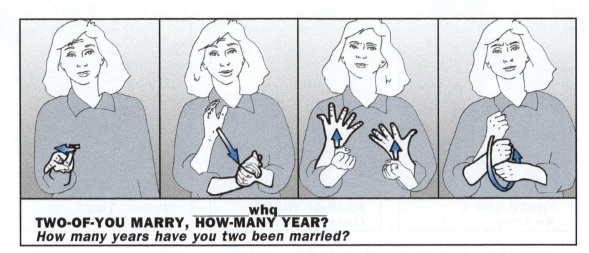

whq
TWO-OF-YOU MARRY, HOW-MANY YEAR?
How many years have you two been married?

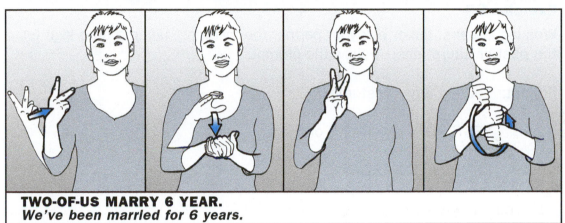

TWO-OF-US MARRY 6 YEAR.
We've been married for 6 years.

Grammar Note

Some personal pronouns can incorporate number as in TWO-OF-YOU and TWO-OF-US above. Another form incorporating the number 2 is:

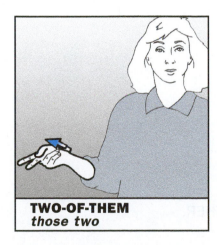

TWO-OF-THEM
those two

8

The numbers 3, 4, and 5 can also be incorporated into some personal pronouns, but they have a circular movement. Numbers greater than 5 cannot be incorporated. Some examples are:

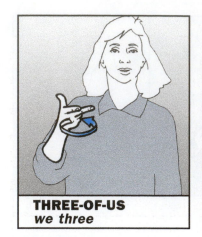

THREE-OF-US
we three

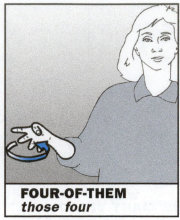

FOUR-OF-THEM
those four

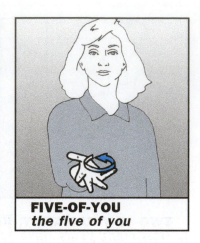

FIVE-OF-YOU
the five of you

Exercise 8B

Working in pairs, tell or ask your partner the following, using a time sign for the past or future tense. Follow the prompt.

Prompt: You – marry – yesterday.

       YESTERDAY I MARRY I. or

       I MARRY YESTERDAY I.

1. You – marry – will.
2. He/She – marry – will?
3. You – birthday – tomorrow.
4. The three of them – come – later?
5. He/She – birthday – recently?
6. You – before – marry?
7. The two of you – meet – a long time ago.
8. You – marry – in the distant future.
9. You – go – after awhile.
10. The two of you – take test – before?

FRIENDS AND ACQUAINTANCES

             _____q_____
Chris: YESTERDAY I SEE YOU. WITH FRIEND?

Lisa: TWO-OF-US GOOD-FRIEND GROW-UP-TOGETHER.

     _____q_____
Chris: BOYFRIEND?

Lisa: (gestures, no) FRIEND FINISH.

Chris: OH-I-SEE. LOOK-LIKE YOU-TWO GOING-TOGETHER. I WRONG I.

Key Structures

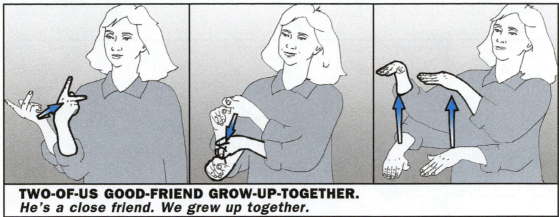

TWO-OF-US GOOD-FRIEND GROW-UP-TOGETHER.
He's a close friend. We grew up together.

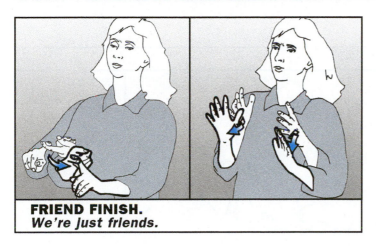

FRIEND FINISH.
We're just friends.

Note

FINISH is used in several ways:

1. To indicate the extent or limit of something such as in "We're just friends" in the sentence FRIEND FINISH above, or as in the following sentence. (Note that the movement is a repeated one.)

8

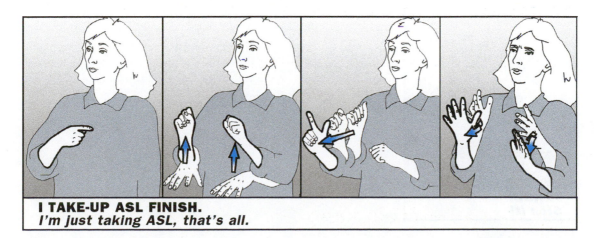

I TAKE-UP ASL FINISH.
I'm just taking ASL, that's all.

2. Before or after the verb to show an action is completed or has been done, as in the following:

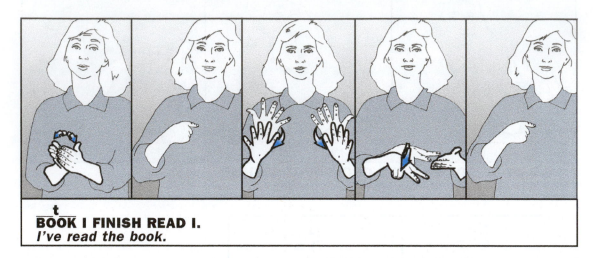

‾‾t‾
BOOK I FINISH READ I.
I've read the book.

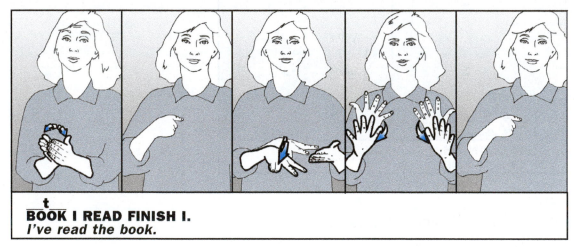

‾‾t‾
BOOK I READ FINISH I.
I've read the book.

3. By itself to mean the following. (Note that there is a single sharp movement.)

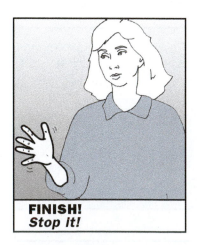

FINISH!
Stop it!

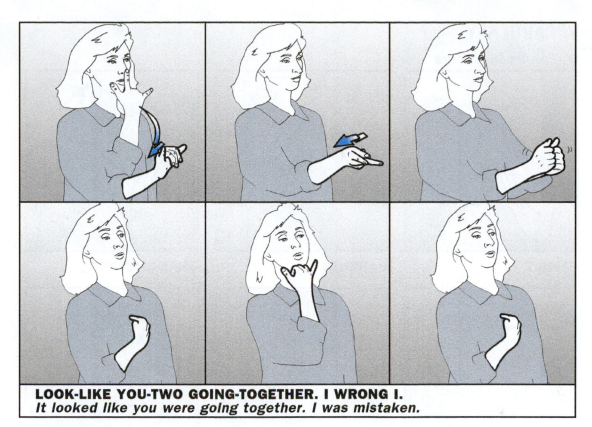

LOOK-LIKE YOU-TWO GOING-TOGETHER. I WRONG I.
It looked like you were going together. I was mistaken.

Exercise 8C

Working in pairs, tell your partner that you have completed the following actions. Follow the prompt.

Prompt: Seen your friend.

___t___
FRIEND I SEE FINISH I. or

___t___
FRIEND I FINISH SEE I.

1. seen the movie
2. visited your grandmother
3. read your ASL book
4. sent the letter
5. gave him/her the book
6. turned on the television
7. gotten married
8. gotten divorced
9. washed clothes
10. passed the test

8

VOCABULARY

▶ Family Members

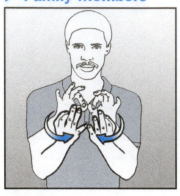

FAMILY

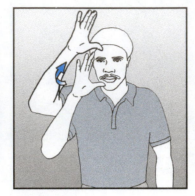

PARENTS

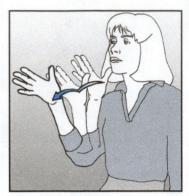

GRANDMOTHER

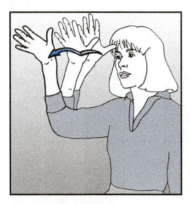

GRANDFATHER

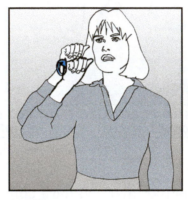

AUNT

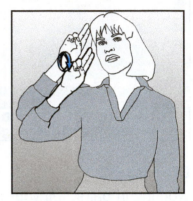

UNCLE

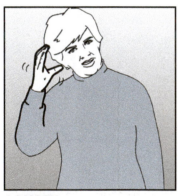

COUSIN

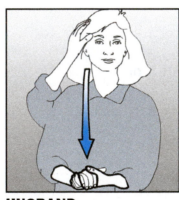

HUSBAND

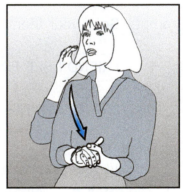

WIFE

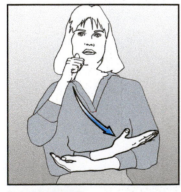

DAUGHTER

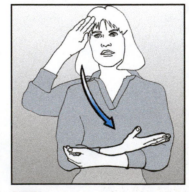

SON

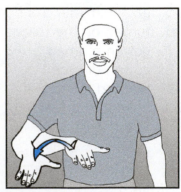

CHILDREN

▶ **Relationships**

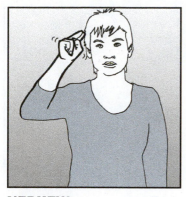

NEPHEW

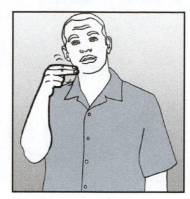

NIECE

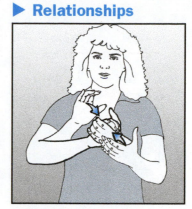

MARRY, marriage

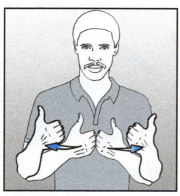

SEPARATED, separate

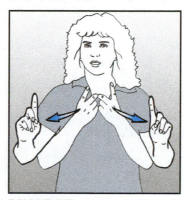

DIVORCE

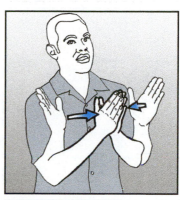

BACK-TOGETHER, reconciled

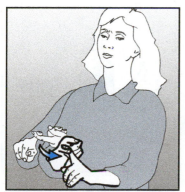

FRIEND

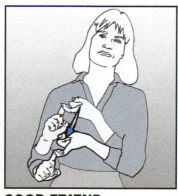

GOOD-FRIEND

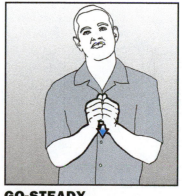

GO-STEADY, go together, dating

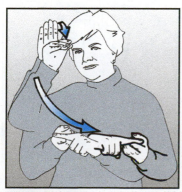

BOYFRIEND

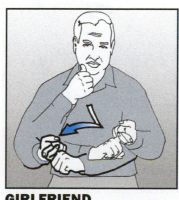

GIRLFRIEND

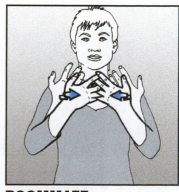

ROOMMATE

8

▶ Tense Indicators

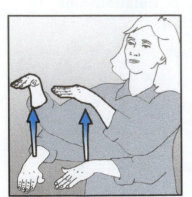

GROW-UP-TOGETHER

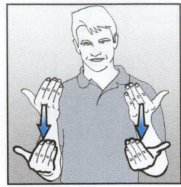

NOW, today, present

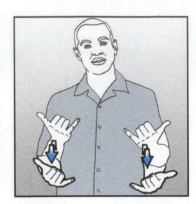

TODAY

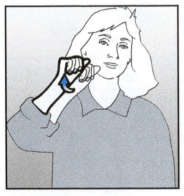

YESTERDAY, past

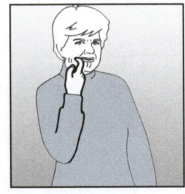

RECENT, recently

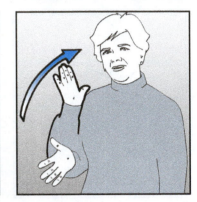

LONG-AGO

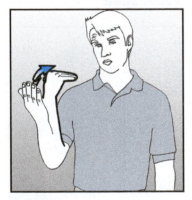

BEFORE

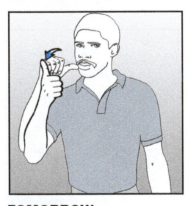

TOMORROW

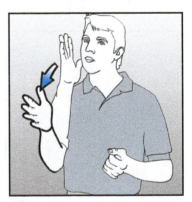

WILL, future

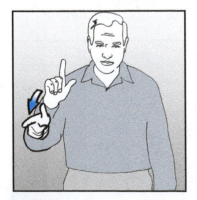

LATER

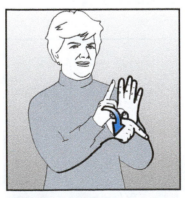

AFTER-AWHILE

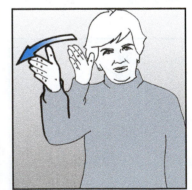

FAR-IN-FUTURE

▶ **Other Vocabulary**

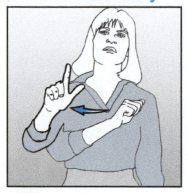

#ALL

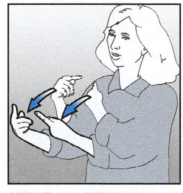

SINCE, up till now

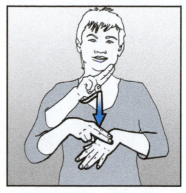

OF-COURSE, naturally

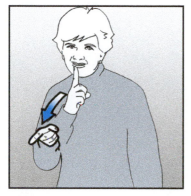

REALLY

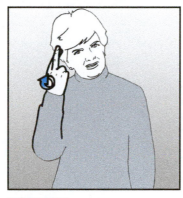

REALIZE, reason

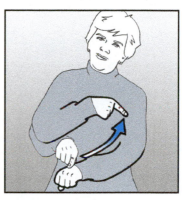

LONG, lengthy

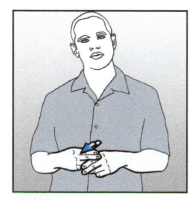

SHORT

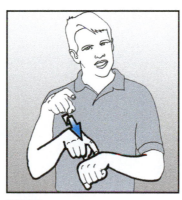

TIME

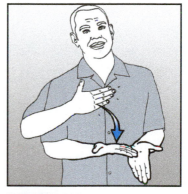

BIRTHDAY

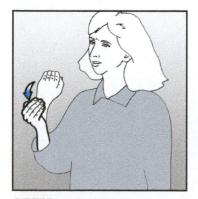

SEEM, appears

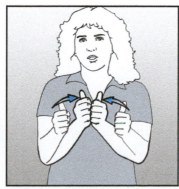

WITH, together

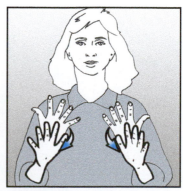

FINISH

8

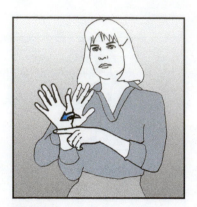

MOVIE

UNIT 9

More Descriptions

In this unit, you will learn how to give descriptions.

You will see several ways to sign to someone without others seeing what you are signing.

You will also learn how to indicate age and time of day, and you will learn more classifiers that indicate size and shape.

In a culture note, you will learn about schools for Deaf children.

HOW OTHERS LOOK

Pat: <u>_____q_____</u>
SEE THERE WOMAN? BEAUTIFUL SHE.

Lisa: <u>_____q_____</u>
KNOW WHO SHE?

Pat: NO. DON'T-KNOW.

Lisa: YOU KNOW SHE. SHE M-A-R-I-A SHE.

Pat: <u>_____q_____</u>
REALLY! THAT-ONE THERE? I SEE SHE BEFORE OLD-5.

SHORT, CHUBBY. NOW CHANGE. I CL:55-EYES-FALL-OUT

Key Structures

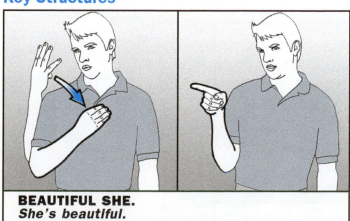

BEAUTIFUL SHE.
She's beautiful.

Note

There are several ways to sign to someone when you do not want others to see what you are saying. Among them are:

1. The signing movement is smaller and closer to the body. Also, the body may be turned slightly to the side.

2. Signing may be done with only one hand while the other hand shields it from view.

3. The information can be fingerspelled close to the body and behind the other hand.

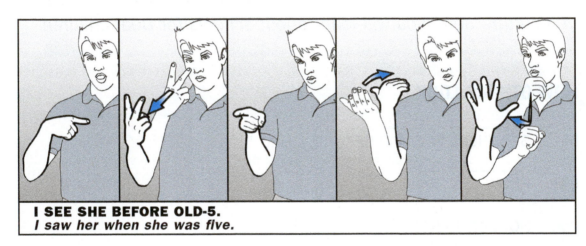

I SEE SHE BEFORE OLD-5.
I saw her when she was five.

Grammar Note

When indicating age, the sign OLD is followed by a number sign. For the numbers 1–5 the palm is turned outward as in OLD-5 above.

When indicating time of day, the sign TIME is followed by a number sign for the hour (and minute). As with indicating age, the palm is also turned outward for the numbers 1–5 as in the following two sentences:

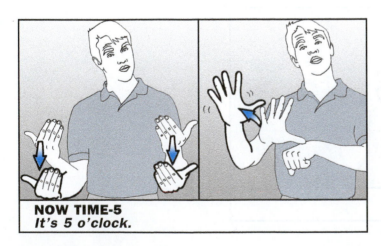

NOW TIME-5
It's 5 o'clock.

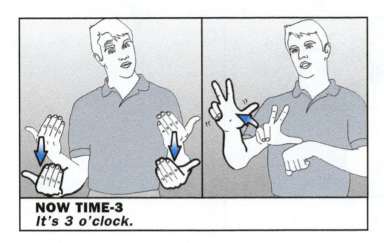

NOW TIME-3
It's 3 o'clock.

However, when indicating a count, the palm is turned inward for the numbers 1–5. Note also, the number can precede or follow the noun as in the following two sentences:

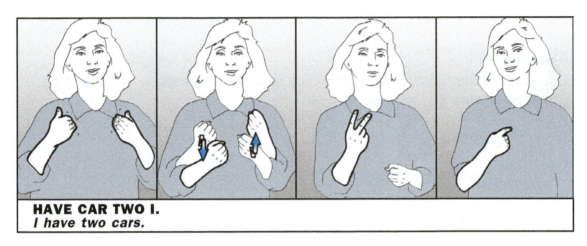

HAVE CAR TWO I.
I have two cars.

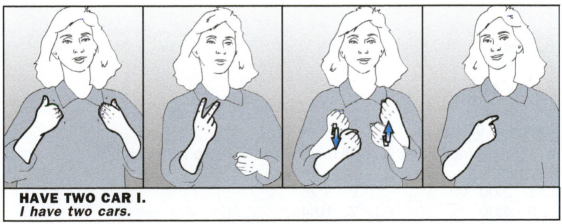

HAVE TWO CAR I.
I have two cars.

9

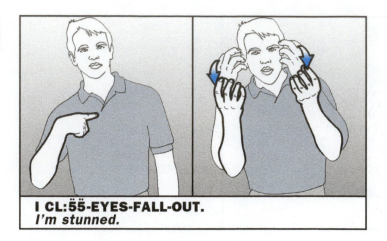

I CL:55̈-EYES-FALL-OUT.
I'm stunned.

Note

Classifiers are often used humorously as in the sentence above in which the classifier 5̈5̈ representing "small, round objects" (see Unit 7) is used to describe an improbable event.

Exercise 9A

Use each of the following in a sentence describing someone or something you know. Follow the prompt.

Prompt: beautiful

      MY MOTHER BEAUTIFUL.

1. good looking
2. slim
3. ugly
4. cute
5. pretty
6. thin
7. chubby

Exercise 9B

a. Tell your friend that you will meet him/her at the following times:

1. 2:00	6. 3:25
2. 4:00	7. 10:45
3. 11:00	8. 5:15
4. 1:30	9. 11:15
5. 12:30	10. 2:10

b. Tell your friend that your brother or sister is the following ages:

1. 7 years	3. 9 years	5. 18 years	7. 4 years
2. 3 years	4. 5 years	6. 21 years	8. 6 years

PERSONALITY

Alex: J-O-H-N HE STUBBORN HE.

Pat: I KNOW^THAT. I REMEMBER TWO-OF-US SMALL THERE SCHOOL-FOR-DEAF. WEEKEND J-O-H-N DON'T-WANT GO-AWAY HOME. WANT STAY SCHOOL-FOR-DEAF. PARENTS PULL. HE STUBBORN, WON'T GO. PARENTS GIVE-UP. J-O-H-N STAY PLAY. HE MISCHIEVOUS HE WOW.

Alex: STILL MISCHIEVOUS.

Key Structures

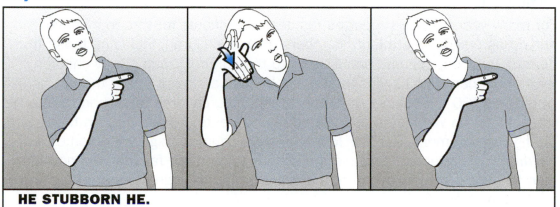

HE STUBBORN HE.
He was stubborn.

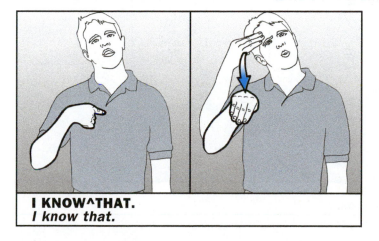

I KNOW^THAT.
I know that.

Note

Note the contraction of KNOW and THAT as indicated by the symbol "^" in KNOW^THAT above.

9

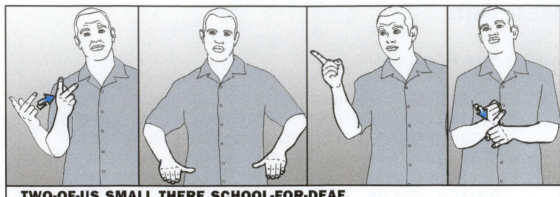

TWO-OF-US SMALL THERE SCHOOL-FOR-DEAF.
We were in the school for Deaf children together when we were small.

Culture Note

For many years, state supported residential "schools for the deaf" have served as places where large numbers of Deaf children, including those from hearing families, become socialized into the cultural group. Many children learn American Sign Language at schools such as these rather than at home. Until the 1960's, because of distance and cost, children often had to stay at the schools on weekends and visited their parents' homes only on holidays or during the summers. But like John in the dialogue on page 115, some Deaf children were reluctant to leave the school. When their families did not use sign language, the attraction of the school, with its large number of signers, was often stronger.

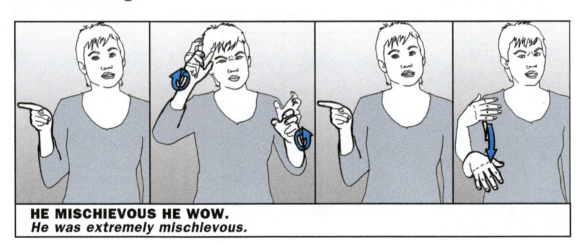

HE MISCHIEVOUS HE WOW.
He was extremely mischievous.

Exercise 9C

Use each of the following traits in a sentence describing someone you know:

1. dumb
2. smart
3. mischievous
4. stubborn
5. friendly
6. stuck-up
7. sweet-natured
8. soft-hearted
9. odd
10. crazy

PHYSICAL FEATURES

Lisa: I LOOK-FOR MAN, NAME SLIP-MIND, TALL, EYEGLASSES,

_____q_____
CL:B̈-POTBELLY. KNOW WHO YOU?

Pat: DON'T-KNOW WHO.

Lisa: BROAD-SHOULDERS, HAVE MUSTACHE.

Pat: OH-I-SEE. I THINK FINISH GO-AWAY.

Lisa: OH-GEE!

Key Structures

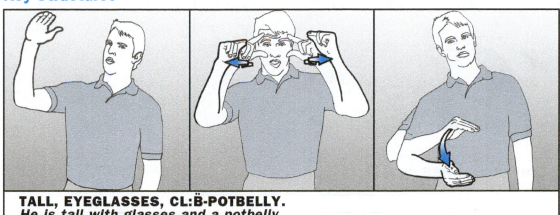

TALL, EYEGLASSES, CL:B̈-POTBELLY.
He is tall with glasses and a potbelly.

Grammar Note

The arc of the movement of the classifier B̈ can vary to indicate smaller and larger sizes, piles, or amounts of something. Compare the following to CL:B̈-POTBELLY:

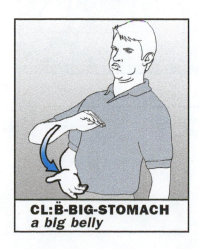

CL:B̈-BIG-STOMACH
a big belly

9

Some other examples of the use of CL:B̈ are:

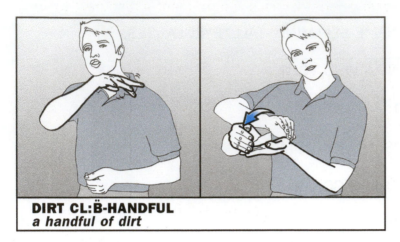

DIRT CL:B̈-HANDFUL
a handful of dirt

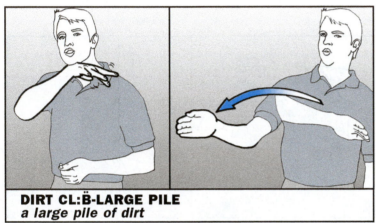

DIRT CL:B̈-LARGE PILE
a large pile of dirt

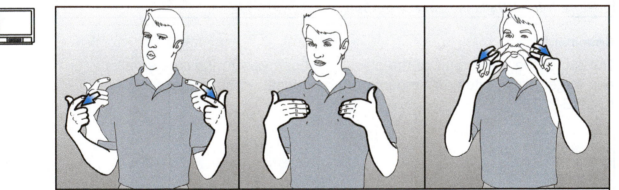

BROAD-SHOULDERS, HAVE MUSTACHE.
He has broad shoulders and a mustache.

Exercise 9D

Describe the following people or characters to the student sitting next to you.

1. a woman with bangs
2. a little girl with a mischievous look
3. a man with broad shoulders
4. a man with a mustache
5. a man with a beer gut
6. a man who is old
7. a woman who is young
8. a man who is good-looking
9. a boy who is cute
10. a woman with glasses

VOCABULARY

▶ Personality Traits

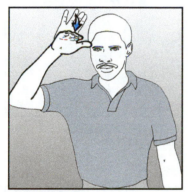

STUBBORN

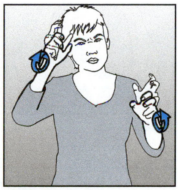

MISCHIEVOUS, mischief

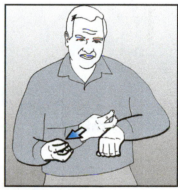

TOUGH, rude, blunt

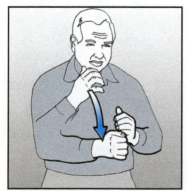

CRUEL, mean

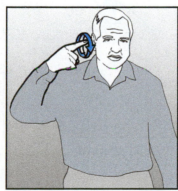

CRAZY

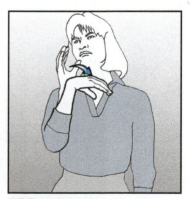

ODD, strange

9

▶ Physical Characteristics

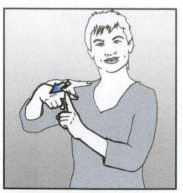

POSITIVE, upbeat, optimistic

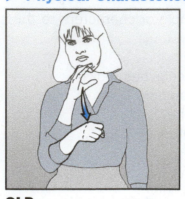

OLD

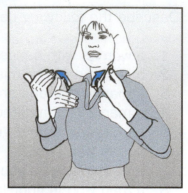

YOUNG

▶ Looks

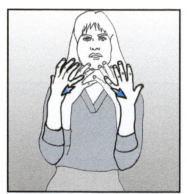

CHUBBY, fat, obese

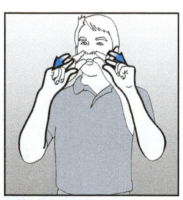

MUSTACHE

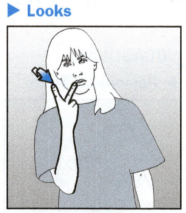

GOOD-LOOKING, handsome

▶ Intelligence

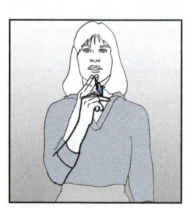

CUTE

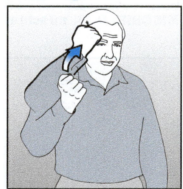

DUMB, stupid

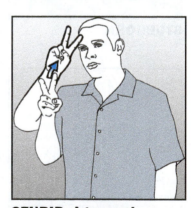

STUPID, ignorant

▶ Noun-Verb Pairs

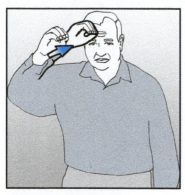

**KNOW-NOTHING,
ignorant, uninformed**

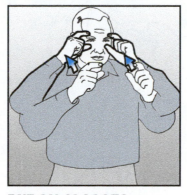

**PUT-ON-GLASSES,
Noun: EYEGLASSES**

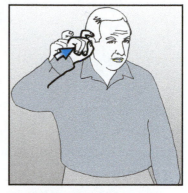

**PUT-ON-HEARING-AID,
Noun: HEARING-AID**

▶ Other Vocabulary

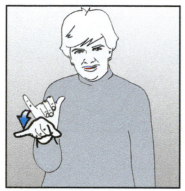

THAT-ONE

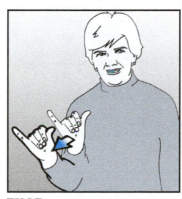

THAT

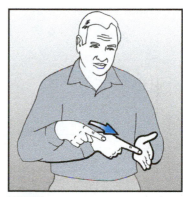

THIS

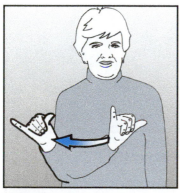

THESE

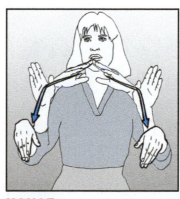

HOUSE

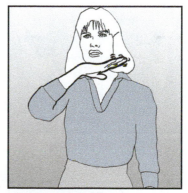

DIRT, dirty

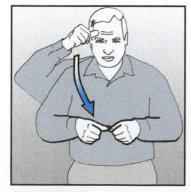

REMEMBER, recall

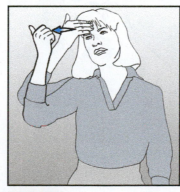

FORGET

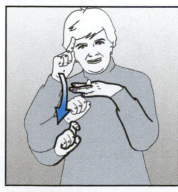

SLIP-MIND

9

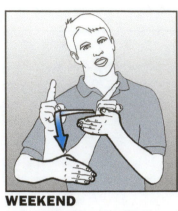

WEEKEND

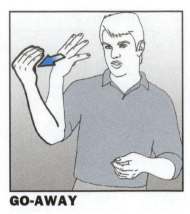

GO-AWAY

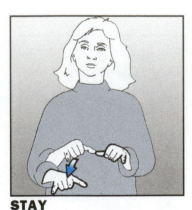

STAY

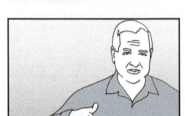

STILL

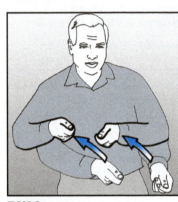

PULL

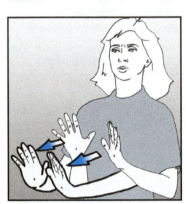

PUSH

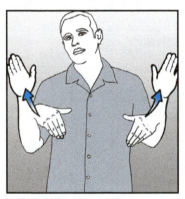

GIVE-UP, sacrifice

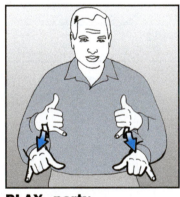

PLAY, party

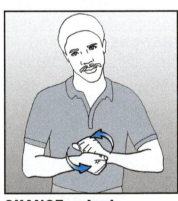

CHANGE, adapt, convert

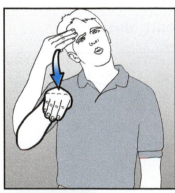

KNOW^THAT

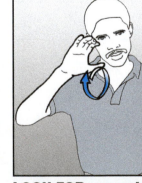

LOOK-FOR, search

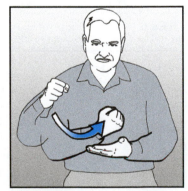

OH-GEE

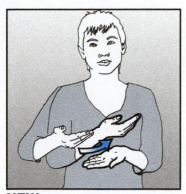

NEW

9

UNIT 10

At Home and Daily Living

In this unit, you will talk about your home and the objects in your home.

You will learn about verbs that change their direction to indicate the subject and object.

You will also learn about classifiers which represent a category and how to add movement to classifiers to show action. In addition, you will learn more classifiers of size and shape.

And you will learn how to indicate regularity, as in "every morning" or "every Sunday."

YOUR RESIDENCE

Alex: RECENT I MOVE-THERE NEW HOUSE. 3 BED+ROOM, 2 BATHROOM, FORMAL+ROOM, KITCHEN. I LIKE.

                    _____q_____

Pat: YOURSELF CARRY-THERE FURNITURE?

Alex: YES. I BORROW TRUCK. CL:3-BACK-UP. LOAD-UP. DRIVE-TO

                          when

      NEW HOUSE. UNLOAD. FINISH I CL:∧-FALL-ON-BACK TIRED.

Key Structures

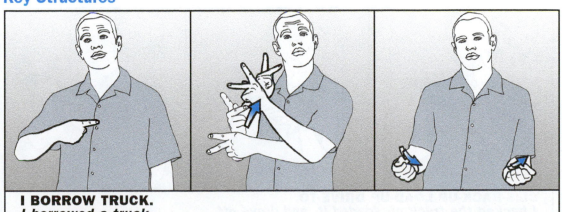

I BORROW TRUCK.
I borrowed a truck.

Grammar Note

Unit 3 includes examples of verbs which change the direction of their movement to indicate the subject and object (HELP, GIVE, SEND, TELL, SHOW, LOOK-AT, PAY).

BORROW, TAKE, SUMMON, CHOOSE and other verbs also change the direction of their movement to indicate subject and object. However, the movement for showing subject and object is the reverse of the verbs in Unit 3. Compare the movements of GIVE and CHOOSE:

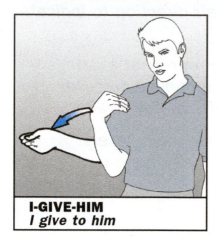

I-GIVE-HIM
I give to him

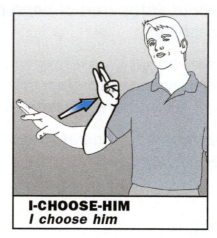

I-CHOOSE-HIM
I choose him

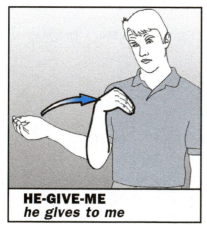

HE-GIVE-ME
he gives to me

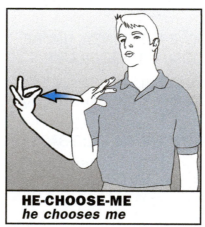

HE-CHOOSE-ME
he chooses me

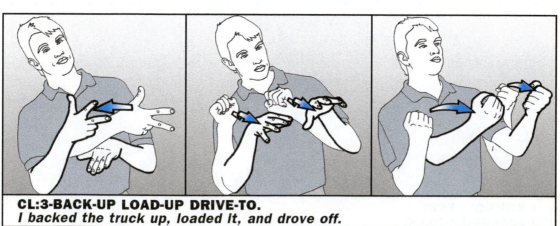

CL:3-BACK-UP LOAD-UP DRIVE-TO.
I backed the truck up, loaded it, and drove off.

Grammar Note

Some predicates have classifier handshapes which represent a category. CL:3 on page 126, for example, represents a category of vehicles including cars, trucks, trains, bicycles, and boats. These classifiers do not indicate size or shape like the classifiers presented in earlier units. Some other classifier handshapes which represent categories are:

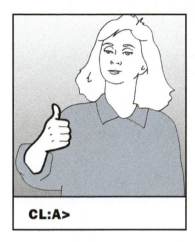

CL:A>

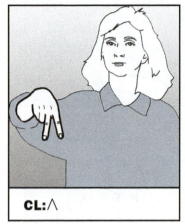

CL:∧

Objects which do not move such as a house or other building, a statue.

Person standing upright or an animal which stands upright such as an ape.

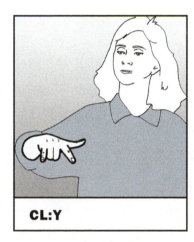

CL:Y

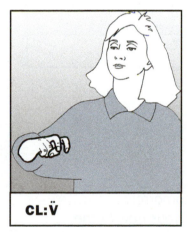

CL:V̈

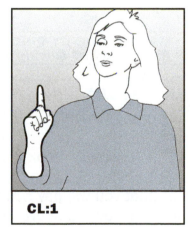

CL:1

Aircraft with wings (not helicopters or rockets).

A crouched or sitting person or animal.

An upright person or animal such as a bear walking on its hind legs.

10

The movement of these classifiers can indicate the action of the predicate as in CL:3-BACK-UP in the sentence above or the manner as in:

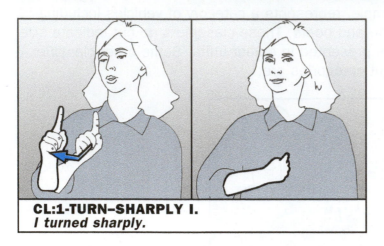

CL:1-TURN–SHARPLY I.
I turned sharply.

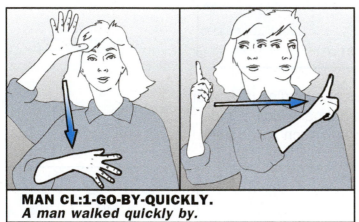

MAN CL:1-GO-BY-QUICKLY.
A man walked quickly by.

Exercise 10A

Ask or tell your friend:

1. to choose a book
2. to help you cook
3. that you will pay him tomorrow
4. that you will show her your new home
5. if you can borrow her car
6. that you will summon a doctor
7. to choose the pink shoes
8. if you can take his book
9. to summon your mother
10. that she can take your magazine

Exercise 10B

Use a classifier predicate to show the following:

1. a woman slipped on the ice and fell
2. a man walking by leisurely
3. a building just standing there
4. a boy standing looking at you
5. a crouched cat
6. three airplanes sitting side by side on the runway
7. a bus zooming by
8. a car going over a bumpy road

OBJECTS IN YOUR RESIDENCE

Alex: HOUSE NEW, BIG, HAVE TWO FLOOR++. BED+ROOM UPSTAIRS, BASEMENT DOWN. DINING+ROOM WINDOW BIG CL:11-SQUARE-SHAPE TABLE CL:B-THERE, SUNSHINE.

Pat: FAMILY+ROOM?

Alex: YES. MY FAVORITE. CHAIR CL:CC⇒-LONG-THERE T-V CL:A>-THERE. I SIT LOOK-AT.

Pat: WOW NICE.

Key Structures

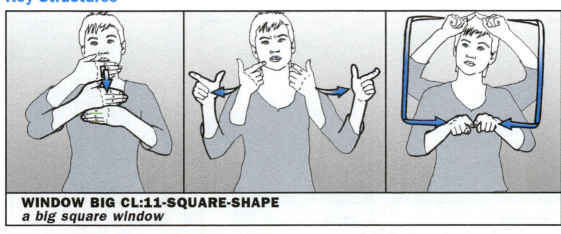

WINDOW BIG CL:11-SQUARE-SHAPE
a big square window

10

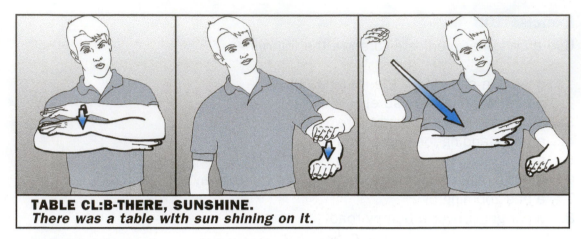

TABLE CL:B-THERE, SUNSHINE.
There was a table with sun shining on it.

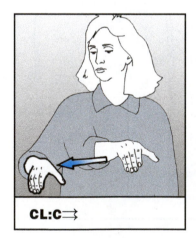

CHAIR CL:CC⇉-LONG-THERE.
There was a sofa.

Grammar Note

The three sentences above all use classifier predicates which specify size and shape. They are:

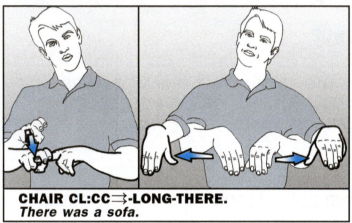

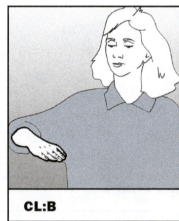

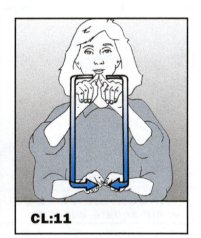

CL:C⇉	CL:B	CL:11
To describe thickish objects such as a sofa, counter, low hedge, or a thick border or edge.	To describe a flat surface or object such as a table top, counter top, or small rug.	To indicate the outline of a shape such as a window.

Note

In the sentence TABLE CL:B-THERE, SUNSHINE, note that the classifier hand-shape, CL:B is held on one hand while the other hand continues the rest of the sentence.

Exercise 10C

Which classifier would you use to indicate the following:

1. a breakfast bar
2. a jogging man
3. a statue in a garden
4. a rectangular swimming pool
5. a truck whizzing by
6. a car coming to an abrupt stop
7. a round swimming pool
8. a wide border of flowers
9. a bath mat on the floor
10. a house

WHAT YOU DO EVERY DAY

                              _____whq_____
Chris: YOU FINISH RETIRE. #DO EVERY DAY?

Pat: I ENJOY TAKE-EASY. EVERY-MORNING I GET-UP READ NEWSPAPER,
       DRINK COFFEE. I NOT EAT BREAKFAST. MOST TIME I OUT LUNCH.
       EVERY-NIGHT I COOK. SOMETIMES GET MOVIE CL:L̈-PUT-IN-DISK,
       LOOK-AT.

                              _____whq_____
Chris: #DO WEEKEND?

Pat: EVERY-SATURDAY I CLEAN-UP HOUSE, WASH-CLOTHES, EVERY-
       SUNDAY I GO-THERE WALK. AFTERNOON REST.

Key Structures

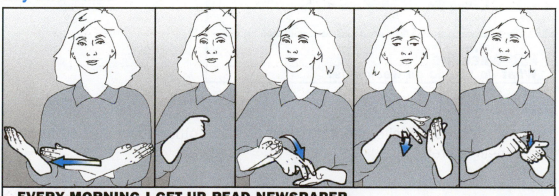

EVERY-MORNING I GET-UP READ NEWSPAPER.
I get up every morning and read the newspaper.

10

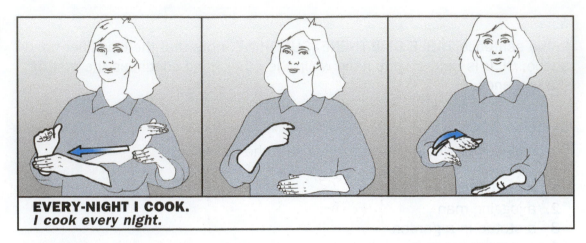

EVERY-NIGHT I COOK.
I cook every night.

Grammar Note

The sweeping movement used in EVERY-MORNING and EVERY-NIGHT above is also used with AFTERNOON to indicate every afternoon:

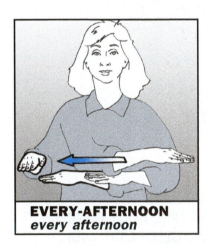

EVERY-AFTERNOON
every afternoon

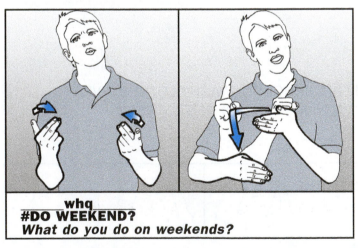

                    whq
#DO WEEKEND?
What do you do on weekends?

Note

In addition to #DO above and #ALL (Unit 8) some other signs derived from fingerspelling are:

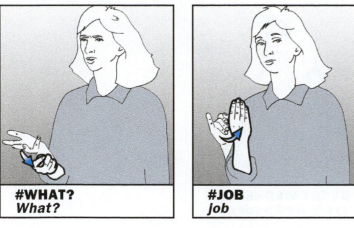

#WHAT?
What?

#JOB
job

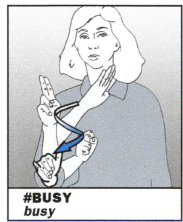

#BUSY
busy

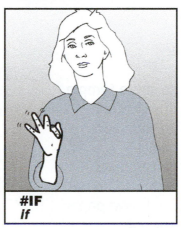

#IF
If

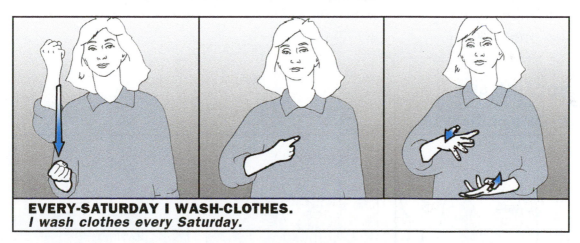

EVERY-SATURDAY I WASH-CLOTHES.
I wash clothes every Saturday.

Grammar Note

The downward continuous movement of EVERY-SATURDAY above can be used with other days of the week as in the examples on the following page.

10

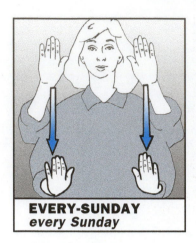

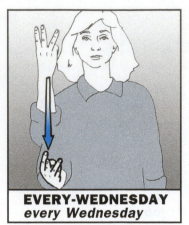

EVERY-SUNDAY
every Sunday

EVERY-WEDNESDAY
every Wednesday

Exercise 10D

Tell your partner what you do:

1.	every Saturday	go there temple
2.	every morning	drink coffee
3.	everyday	go to school
4.	every evening	cook
5.	every Sunday	go to church
6.	every Tuesday	clean up house
7.	every afternoon	read newspaper
8.	every Thursday	eat out
9.	every night	watch TV
10.	every Monday	get flowers

VOCABULARY

▶ Days of the Week

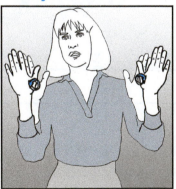

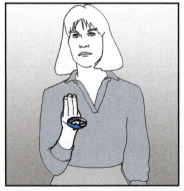

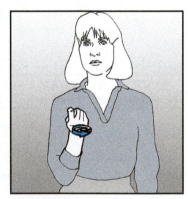

SUNDAY   **MONDAY**   **TUESDAY**

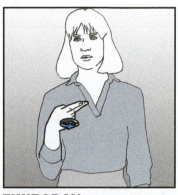

WEDNESDAY

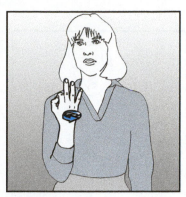

THURSDAY

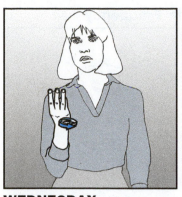

FRIDAY

▶ **Meals, Cooking, and Food**

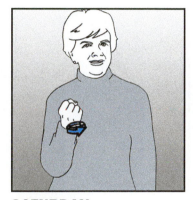

SATURDAY

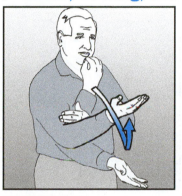

BREAKFAST

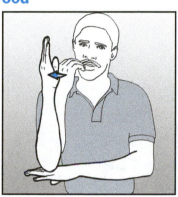

LUNCH

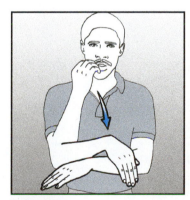

DINNER

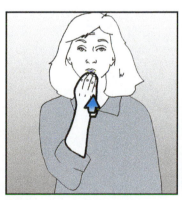

EAT

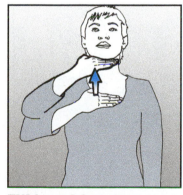

FULL, not hungry

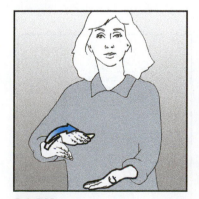

COOK

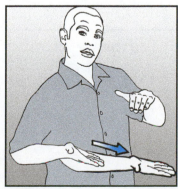

BAKE

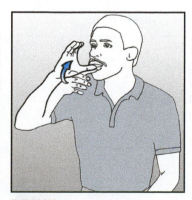

DRINK

10

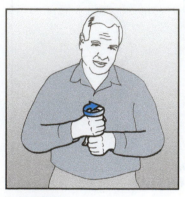

COFFEE

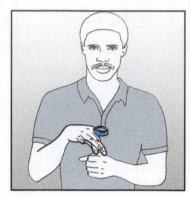

TEA

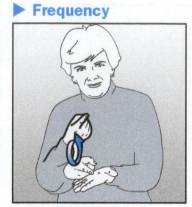

SOMETIMES

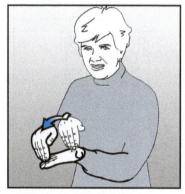

OFTEN, frequently

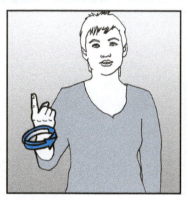

ALWAYS

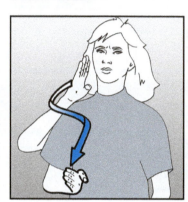

NEVER

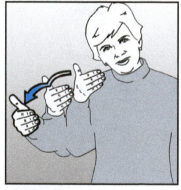

FROM-TIME-TO-TIME

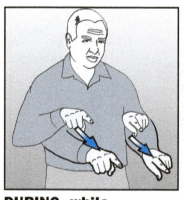

DURING, while

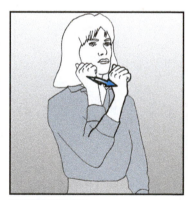

EVERYDAY

▶ **The House**

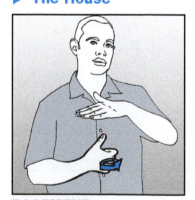

BASEMENT

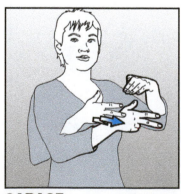

GARAGE

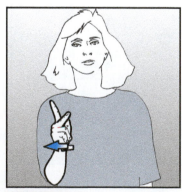

KITCHEN

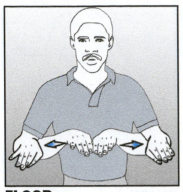

FLOOR

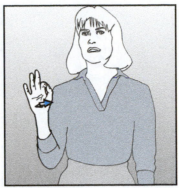

FURNITURE

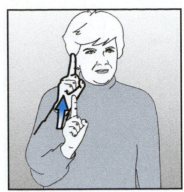

UP, upstairs

▶ **From Fingerspelling**

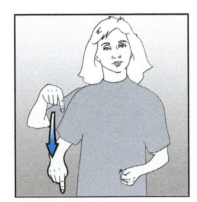

DOWN, downstairs

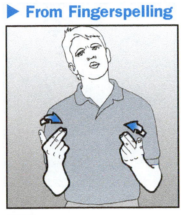

#DO

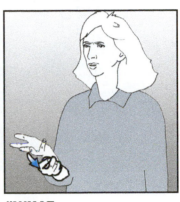

#WHAT

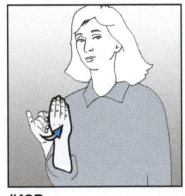

#JOB

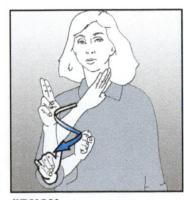

#BUSY

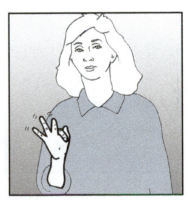

#IF

▶ **Other Vocabulary**

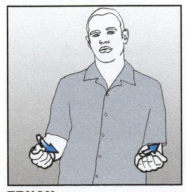

TRUCK

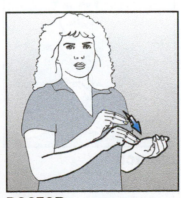

DOCTOR

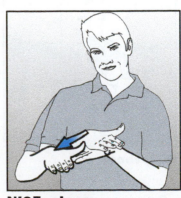

NICE, clean

10

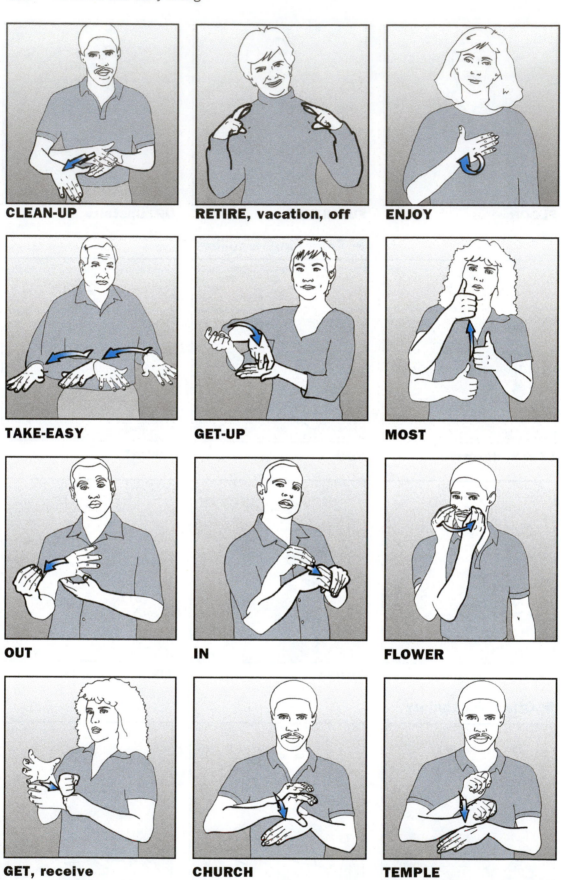

CLEAN-UP

RETIRE, vacation, off

ENJOY

TAKE-EASY

GET-UP

MOST

OUT

IN

FLOWER

GET, receive

CHURCH

TEMPLE

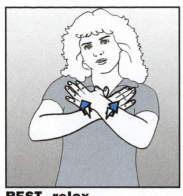

REST, relax

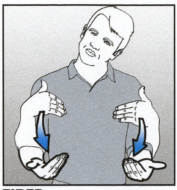

TIRED

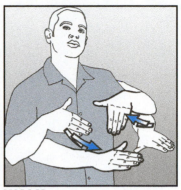

WALK

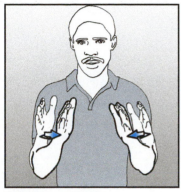

LITTLE, small

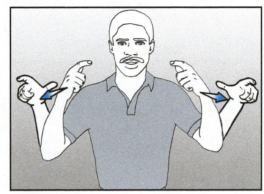

BIG, large

10

UNIT 11

Food and Food Shopping

In this unit, you will talk about food and shopping for food. You will learn how to talk about quantities and prices.

You will learn more classifiers which indicate thickness, width, and depth.

You will also learn to use negative modals such as CAN'T and WON'T, and to use NONE as a negative.

THE MENU

Lisa: $\overline{\quad\quad q\quad\quad}$
TONIGHT #DO?

Chris: COOK WILL I. I THINK #VEG SOUP, CHICKEN, POTATO, SALAD FINISH. PLUS ICE-CREAM.

Lisa: FINE. EASY.

Chris: 1 I THINK-OF. RUN-OUT POTATO, BOTTLE O-I-L DEPLETE.

$\overline{\quad\quad\quad\quad\quad q\quad\quad\quad\quad\quad}$
GO-THERE STORE CAN'T I. NONE TIME. DON'T-MIND YOU GO-THERE?

Lisa: I DON'T-MIND I.

Key Structures

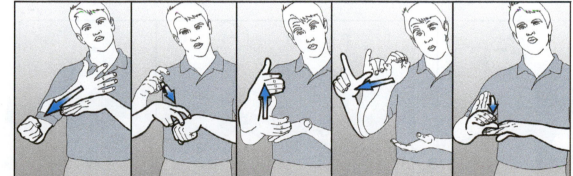

RUN-OUT POTATO, BOTTLE O-I-L DEPLETE.
I'm out of potatoes and oil.

Note

RUN-OUT can be used with most objects such as potatoes, books, paper, and liquids. However, DEPLETE is used to indicate that the contents of a container, usually a liquid, is depleted.

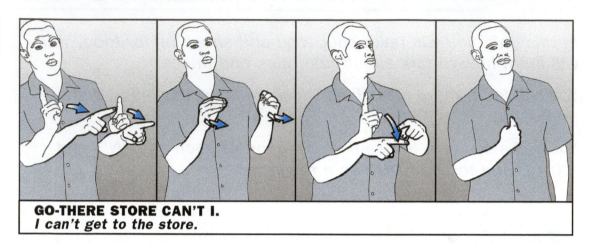

GO-THERE STORE CAN'T I.
I can't get to the store.

Grammar Note

CAN'T and WON'T, negatives of the modals CAN and WILL, are used in the same way as other modals. An example using WON'T is:

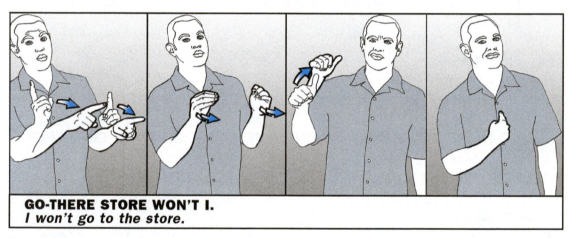

GO-THERE STORE WON'T I.
I won't go to the store.

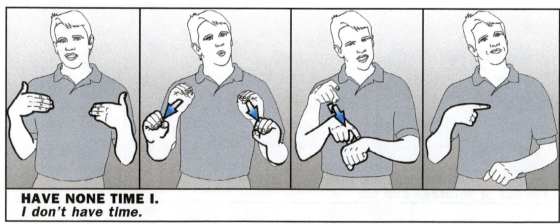

HAVE NONE TIME I.
I don't have time.

Grammar Note

NONE can be used before a noun to indicate an absence or lack of something as in HAVE NONE TIME I on the previous page, or as in the following:

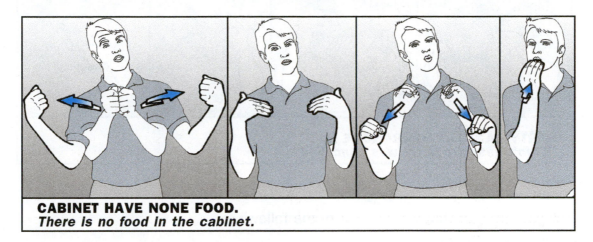

CABINET HAVE NONE FOOD.
There is no food in the cabinet.

Also, NONE can be used with SEE, HEAR, UNDERSTAND as a negative. Note the contractions (^) in the following:

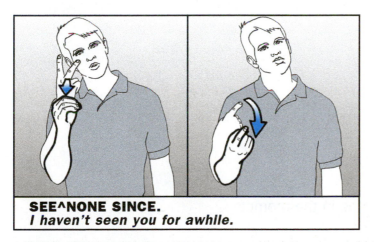

SEE^NONE SINCE.
I haven't seen you for awhile.

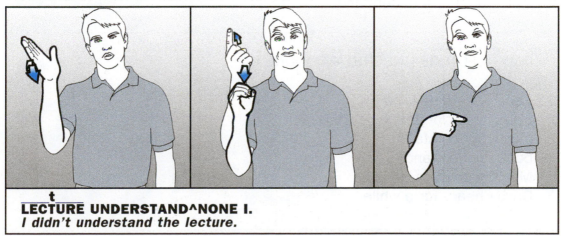

LECTURE UNDERSTAND^NONE I.
I didn't understand the lecture.

11

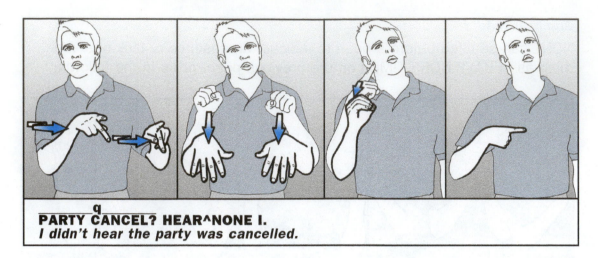

q
PARTY CANCEL? HEAR^NONE I.
I didn't hear the party was cancelled.

Exercise 11A

Tell your partner that you are out of the following:

1. water
2. oranges
3. wine
4. bread
5. cheese
6. milk
7. eggs
8. meat
9. vegetables
10. sugar

Exercise 11B

Use NONE with the following as in the prompt:

Prompt: lecture – understand

         ____t____
        LECTURE UNDERSTAND^NONE I.

1. Bob - see - long time
2. Bob - hear - long time
3. movie - understand
4. book - understand
5. Meg - see - for a while
6. Dave - hear - for a while

QUANTITIES

```
            ____t____
Lisa:   MAKE PIE, I SHOW-YOU.
            ___whq___
Chris:  WHAT PIE?
```

Lisa: C-O-C-O-N-U-T. FIRST, NEED TWO EGG.

Chris: I FINISH BUY 1 D-O-Z.

Lisa: FINE. NEED ONE-HALF L-B BUTTER. 1 CUP MILK. 1 CUP SUGAR.
```
        _____t_____  _____whq_____
Chris:  YOU MAKE PIE, CL:G-THIN O-R CL:G-THICK WHICH?
```

Lisa: LOOK-AT-ME. I-SHOW-YOU.

Key Structures

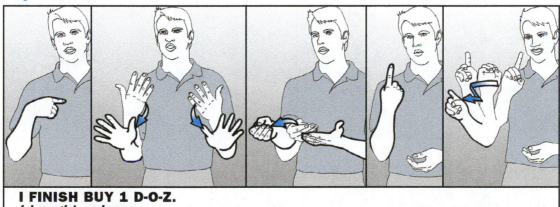

I FINISH BUY 1 D-O-Z.
I bought a dozen.

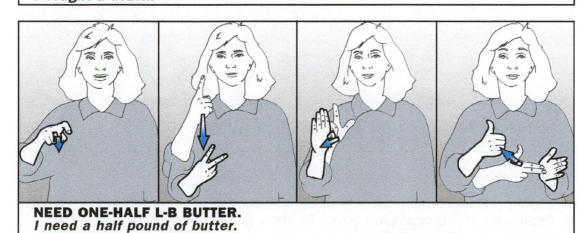

NEED ONE-HALF L-B BUTTER.
I need a half pound of butter.

11

Note

Some abbreviations, used to indicate amounts, such as D-O-Z and L-B are taken from English in the form of fingerspelling. Other examples are:

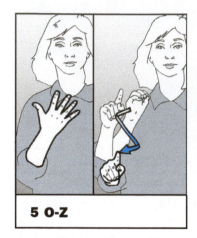

5 O-Z

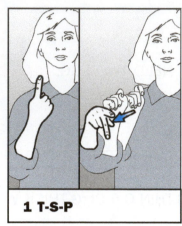

1 T-S-P

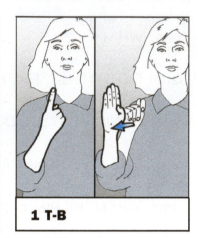

1 T-B

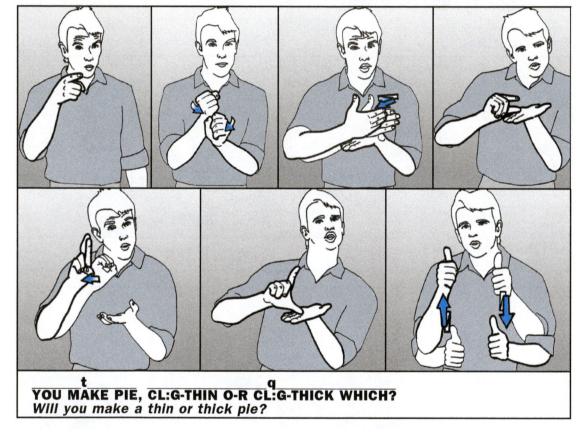

t   q
YOU MAKE PIE, CL:G-THIN O-R CL:G-THICK WHICH?
Will you make a thin or thick pie?

Grammar Note

The classifier handshape CL:G is used to show various thicknesses, widths, or depths as in the example above. To show greater thickness, width, or depth, the classifier CL:BB may be used as in the following:

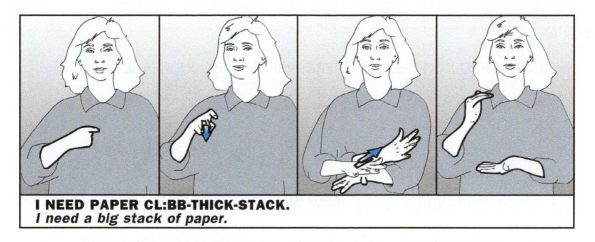

I NEED PAPER CL:BB-THICK-STACK.
I need a big stack of paper.

Movement is combined with CL:G to show a layer of thickness as in:

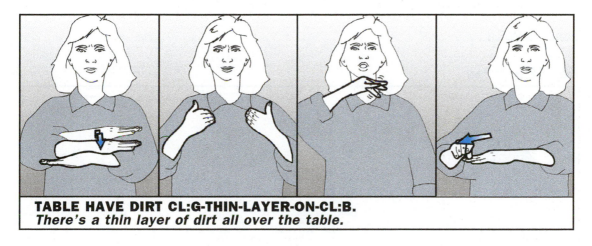

TABLE HAVE DIRT CL:G-THIN-LAYER-ON-CL:B.
There's a thin layer of dirt all over the table.

Exercise 11C

Indicate the thickness, width or depth of the following:

Prompt: PIE CL:G-THIN.

1. a box 12 inches deep
2. water in a glass
3. water in a bucket
4. water on the floor
5. a cut of meat
6. a book
7. a coat
8. a newspaper
9. eyeglasses
10. a stack of paper

11

PRICES

Chris: SHOCKED I. STORE I GO-THERE, PRICE AWFUL INCREASE.

           ____whq____
Lisa: WHAT BUY?

Chris: I BUY APPLE 3, COST 2-DOLLAR, BUTTER 1 L-B, 3-DOLLAR-99,
        ICE-CREAM 1 G-A-L 4-DOLLAR-BLANK.

                    ____whq____
Lisa   WOW, EXPENSIVE. PRICE TOTAL?

Chris: I GO-THERE STORE, HAVE 50 DOLLAR, COME-HERE HOME LEFT
        50-CENT.

Lisa: AWFUL.

Key Structures

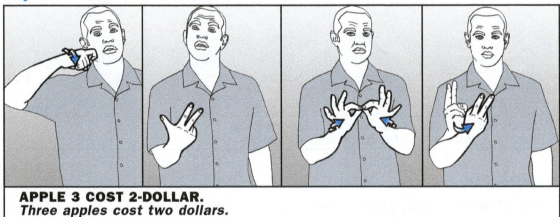

APPLE 3 COST 2-DOLLAR.
Three apples cost two dollars.

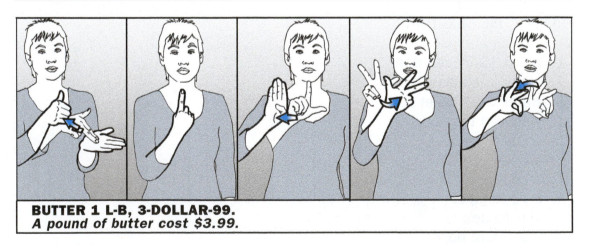

BUTTER 1 L-B, 3-DOLLAR-99.
A pound of butter cost $3.99.

Grammar Note

1-DOLLAR can incorporate the numbers 2–10 only. Numbers higher than 10 are not incorporated as in:

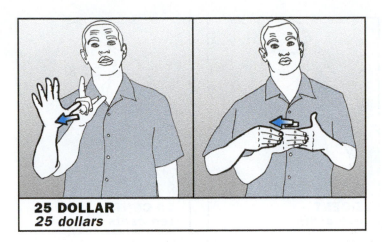

25 DOLLAR
25 dollars

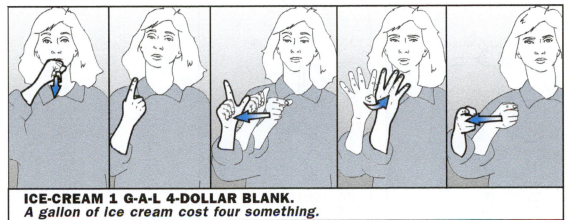

ICE-CREAM 1 G-A-L 4-DOLLAR BLANK.
A gallon of ice cream cost four something.

Note

When the amount is not known to the exact cent, the sign BLANK may be used following the dollar amount to give an approximate amount as in the sentence above.

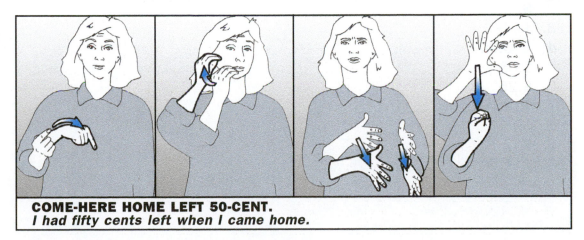

COME-HERE HOME LEFT 50-CENT.
I had fifty cents left when I came home.

Grammar Note

The cent amount for each American coin is incorporated as in the following examples. Note how numbers higher than 9 are incorporated.

11

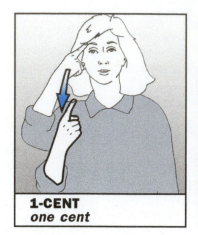

1-CENT
one cent

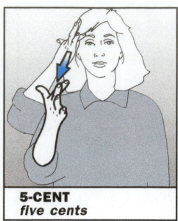

5-CENT
five cents

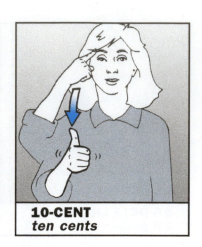

10-CENT
ten cents

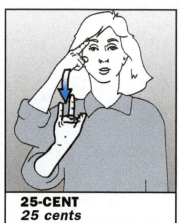

25-CENT
25 cents

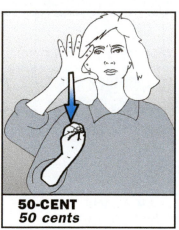

50-CENT
50 cents

Exercise 11D

Indicate the following amounts:

1. $1.98
2. $2.99
3. $4.50
4. $40.00
5. $.05
6. $.25
7. $16.00
8. $9.?
9. $47.?
10. $11.04

VOCABULARY

▶ **Food**

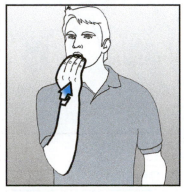

FOOD

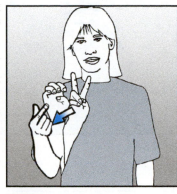

#VEG

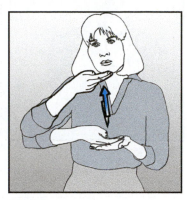

SOUP

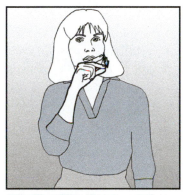

CHICKEN, bird

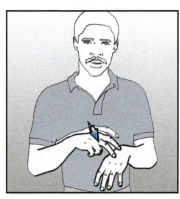

POTATO

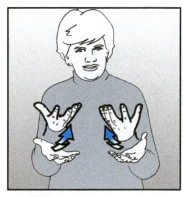

SALAD

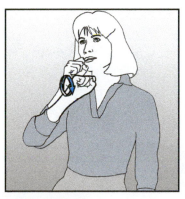

ICE-CREAM

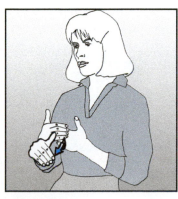

BREAD

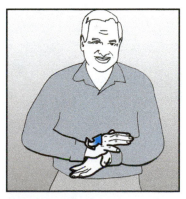

CHEESE

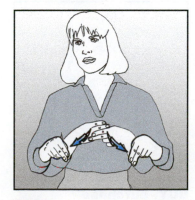

EGG

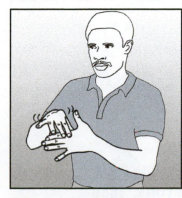

MEAT, beef, steak

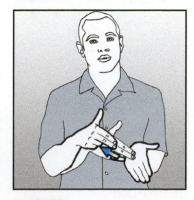

BUTTER

11

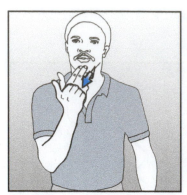

SUGAR

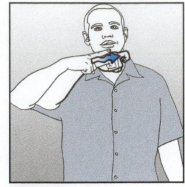

CEREAL

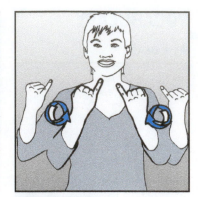

SPAGHETTI

▶ **Drinks**

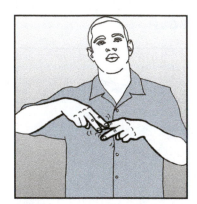

SALT

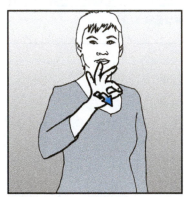

PEPPER

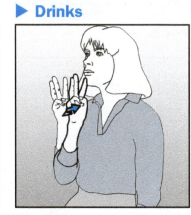

WATER

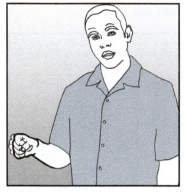

MILK

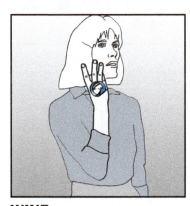

WINE

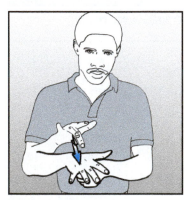

SODA, pop

▶ **Shopping**

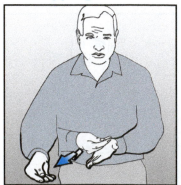

SHOPPING

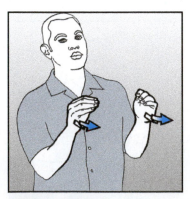

STORE, shop

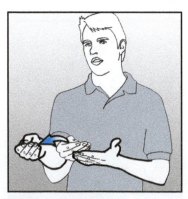

BUY, purchase

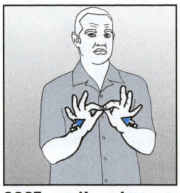

COST, worth, value

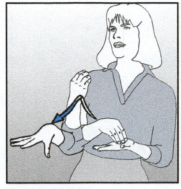

EXPENSIVE

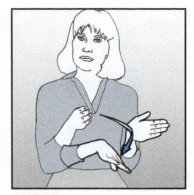

CHEAP

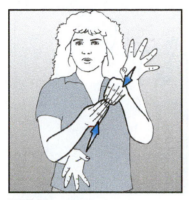

TOTAL, sum

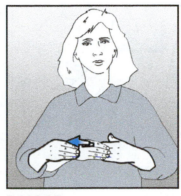

DOLLAR

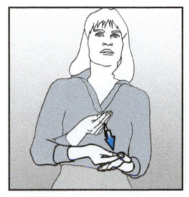

MONEY

▶ **Negatives of Modals**　　　　　　　　　　　　▶ **Other Vocabulary**

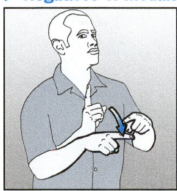

CAN'T

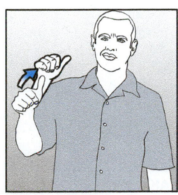

WON'T, refuse

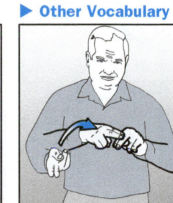

INCREASE

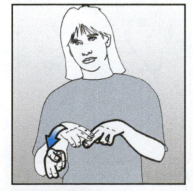

DECREASE

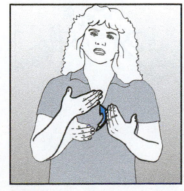

EASY

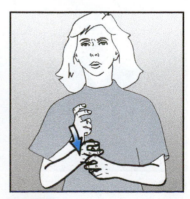

HARD

11

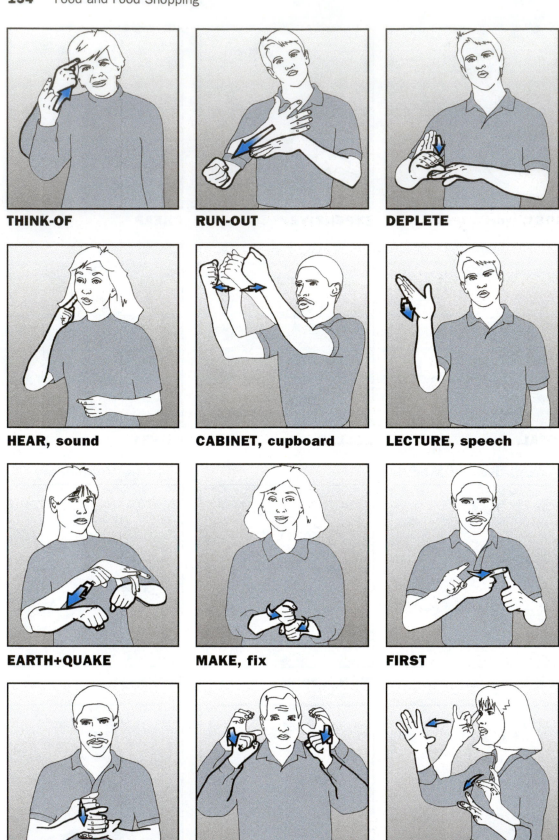

THINK-OF

RUN-OUT

DEPLETE

HEAR, sound

CABINET, cupboard

LECTURE, speech

EARTH+QUAKE

MAKE, fix

FIRST

CUP

SHOCKED

AWFUL, terrible

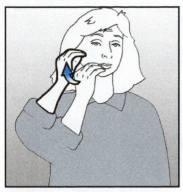

HOME

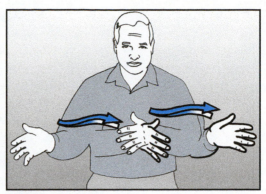

WIND, breeze

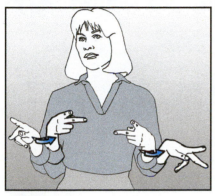

PARTY

11

UNIT 12

Offering and Declining

In this unit, you will learn how to offer and decline politely. You will also learn about explaining why you must decline.

You will learn about offering help, explaining what is wrong, and what you need.

In a culture note, you will learn about telecommunication used by Deaf people.

FOOD AND DRINK

```
        _____q_____
Pat:    WANT EAT?


Alex:   SURE. I NOT-YET EAT ALL-DAY. I HUNGRY I.

                        _____q_____
Pat:    I MAKE SANDWICH. YOU WANT?


Alex:   FINE, ANY.
        _____whq_____                      __whq__
Pat:    DRINK WHAT? HAVE BEER, COKE, WATER WHICH?

                _____q_____
Alex:   COKE THANK-YOU. WANT HELP?
```

Key Structures

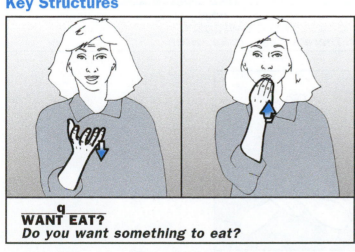

WANT EAT?
Do you want something to eat?

157 12

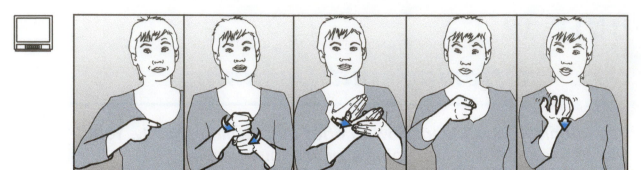

I MAKE SANDWICH. $\overline{\overset{q}{\text{YOU WANT?}}}$
I'm making a sandwich. Do you want one?

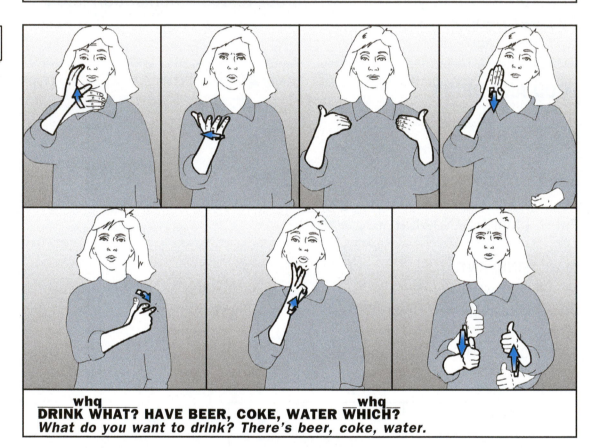

$\overline{\overset{whq}{\text{DRINK WHAT?}}}$ **HAVE BEER, COKE, WATER** $\overline{\overset{whq}{\text{WHICH?}}}$
What do you want to drink? There's beer, coke, water.

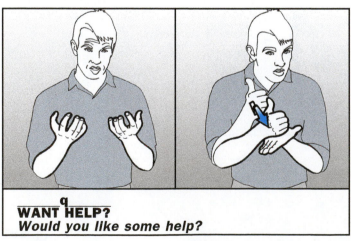

$\overline{\overset{q}{\text{WANT HELP?}}}$
Would you like some help?

Grammar Note

This form of HELP does not show subject or object and is used as a general offer of assistance.

Exercise 12A

Ask your partner if he/she would like:

1. something to drink
2. a coke
3. some help
4. a sandwich
5. a beer
6. some wine
7. some milk
8. something to eat
9. some hot tea
10. some hot chocolate

OFFERING HELP

```
       __t__ _____q_____
Alex:  #TTY, CAN I TYPE TTY-TO-HIM BROTHER? CAR WON'T START.
       I STRUGGLE, GIVE-UP.

       __whq__ _____q_____ _whq__
Pat:   WRONG? MOTOR BREAKDOWN? WHAT?


Alex:  NOT SURE. GAS HAVE. MAYBE BATTERY SHUT-DOWN.

       _____q_____
Pat:   OLD BATTERY?


Alex:  FOUR YEAR.

                          _____q_____
Pat:   I SUSPECT SHUT-DOWN. WANT JUMPSTART?
```

12

Key Structures

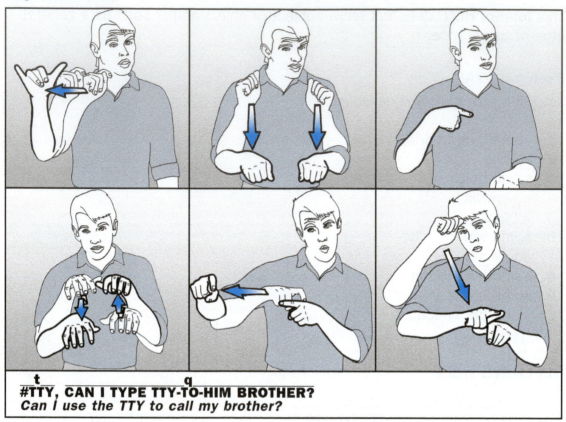

<u>t</u>　　　　　<u>q</u>
#TTY, CAN I TYPE TTY-TO-HIM BROTHER?
Can I use the TTY to call my brother?

Culture Note

A TTY (also called a telecommunications device for the Deaf, a TDD, or teletypewriter) is a device for typing over telephone lines. Anyone having a TTY can call another party who has a TTY. If one of the parties does not have a TTY, there are relay services which one can call via voice or TTY. The relay service will call the other party and relay the conversation between parties as in a normal conversation.

In recent years, more and more Deaf people have been using text pagers with small keyboards for communicating with each other electronically. You may see a Deaf person typing frantically, using his or her thumbs, on one of these pagers. Deaf people are also making heavy use of e-mail.

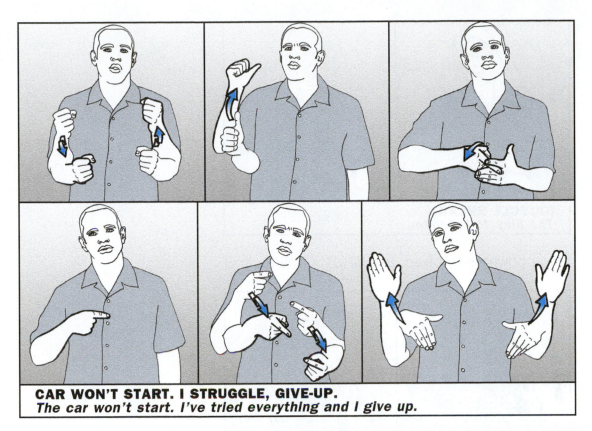

CAR WON'T START. I STRUGGLE, GIVE-UP.
The car won't start. I've tried everything and I give up.

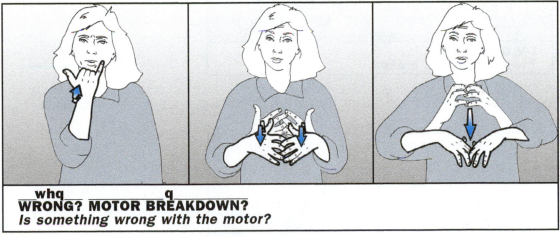

<u>whq</u>   <u>q</u>
WRONG? MOTOR BREAKDOWN?
Is something wrong with the motor?

Note

BREAKDOWN above is used to describe the breakdown of large motors or motor-driven devices. BREAK can be used with most other devices as in:

12

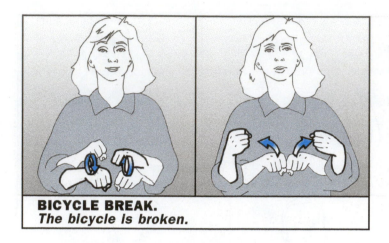

BICYCLE BREAK.
The bicycle is broken.

When power is involved, use SHUTDOWN as in:

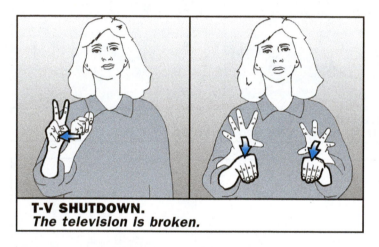

T-V SHUTDOWN.
The television is broken.

When something wears out or burns out, including people, use WEAR-OUT:

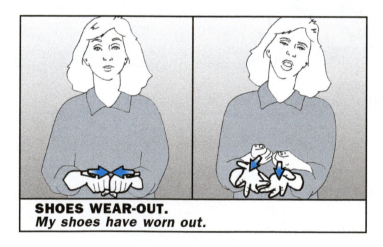

SHOES WEAR-OUT.
My shoes have worn out.

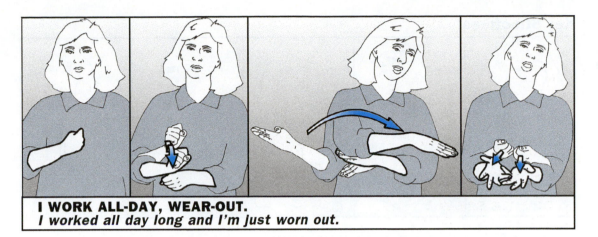

I WORK ALL-DAY, WEAR-OUT.
I worked all day long and I'm just worn out.

Exercise 12B

Indicate to your partner that the following are not working:

1. a computer
2. a typewriter
3. a truck
4. an airplane
5. a TTY
6. a hairdryer
7. a hearing aid
8. a pair of pants
9. a telephone
10. a watch

DECLINING AND EXPLAINING

        _____t_____
Chris: PARTY YOU-INVITE-ME, I MUST DECLINE. CONFLICT.

Alex: ALL-RIGHT. I SAVE FOOD FOR YOU.

Chris: NO. I INCREASE WEIGHT I. I THINK-OF I. I SHOULD BRING-THERE
        whq
        SALAD. #DO?
      ___n___
Alex: WORRY. SELF WILL MAKE.
                 _____q_____
Chris: THANK-YOU. WILL YOU TELL-HER WIFE SORRY?
        ___n___
Alex: SURE. O-K, WORRY.

12

Key Structures

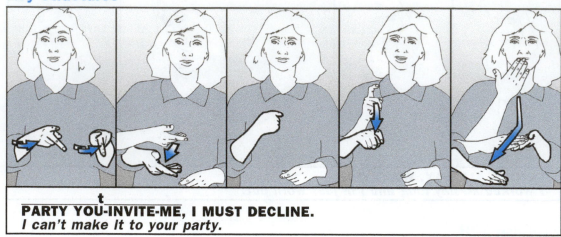

<u>   t   </u>
PARTY YOU-INVITE-ME, I MUST DECLINE.
I can't make it to your party.

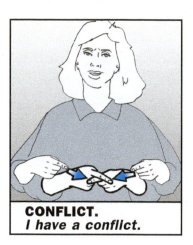

CONFLICT.
I have a conflict.

Grammar Note

Other ways to explain why you must decline include:

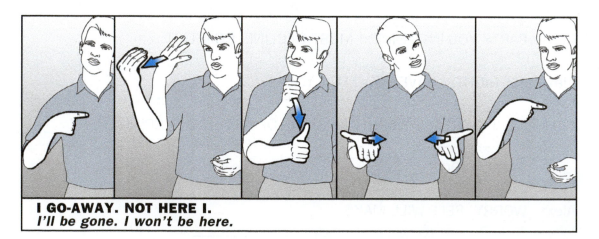

I GO-AWAY. NOT HERE I.
I'll be gone. I won't be here.

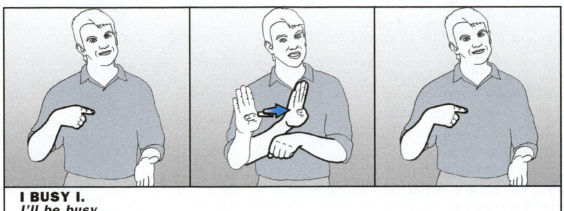

I BUSY I.
I'll be busy.

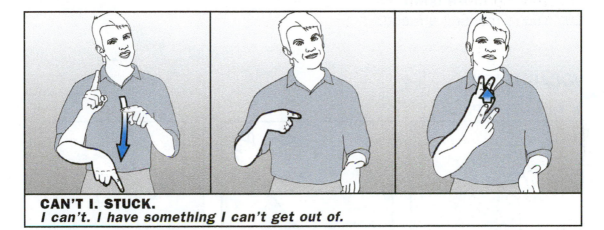

CAN'T I. STUCK.
I can't. I have something I can't get out of.

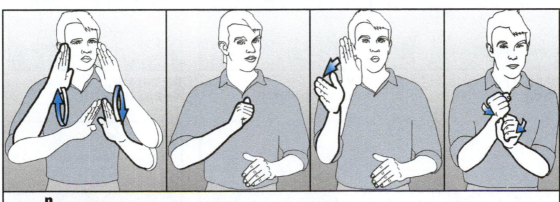

WORRY. SELF WILL MAKE.
Don't worry about it. I'll do it myself.

12

Exercise 12C

Decline an invitation to go out to eat. Give the following explanations:

1. You won't be here.
2. You're busy.
3. You have a conflict.
4. You're stuck.
5. You're sick.
6. You're exhausted.
7. You have to work.
8. You have to study.
9. Your car broke down.
10. You're meeting a friend.

VOCABULARY

▶ **Noun-Verb Pairs**

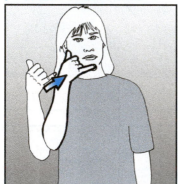

**CALL-BY-PHONE,
Noun: TELEPHONE**

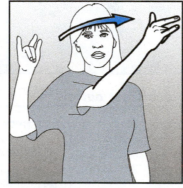

**FLY,
Noun: AIRPLANE**

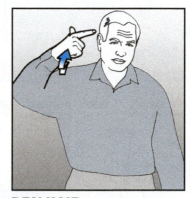

**DRY-HAIR,
Noun: HAIRDRYER**

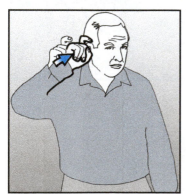

**PUT-ON-HEARING-AID,
Noun: HEARING-AID**

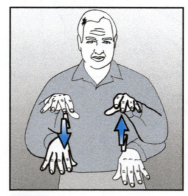

**TYPE,
Noun: TYPEWRITER**

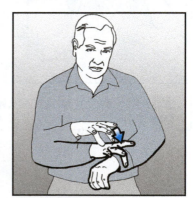

**PUT-ON-WATCH,
Noun: WATCH**

▶ **Food and Drink**

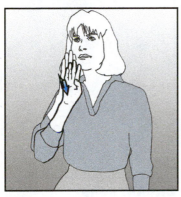

**PUT-IN-GAS,
Noun: GAS**

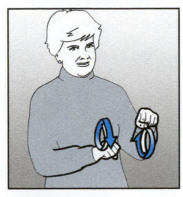

**RIDE-BICYCLE,
Noun: BICYCLE**

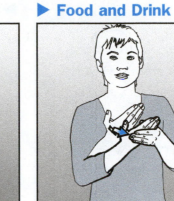

SANDWICH

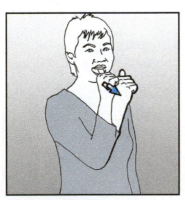

BEER

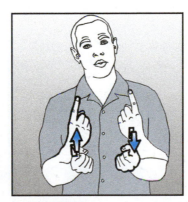

COKE

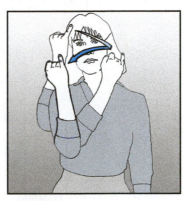

PEPSI

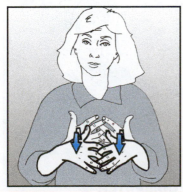

NUTS, peanuts

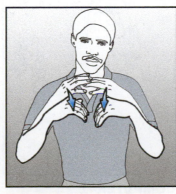

POPCORN

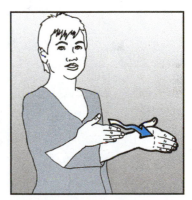

FISH

▶ **Car Trouble**

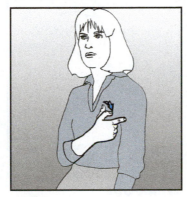

MOTOR, machine, engine

BREAKDOWN, collapse

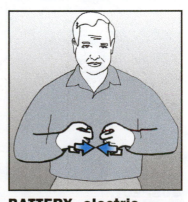

BATTERY, electric

12

▶ **Other Vocabulary**

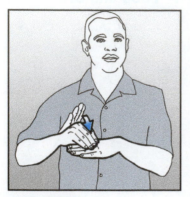

FLAT-TIRE

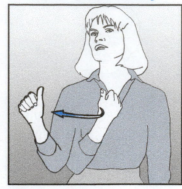

ANY, anything

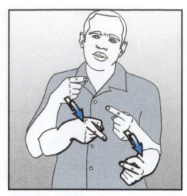

STRUGGLE

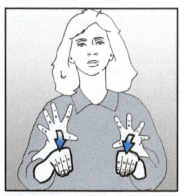

SHUTDOWN, blow out

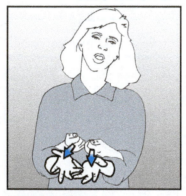

**WEAR-OUT,
burn out, fall apart**

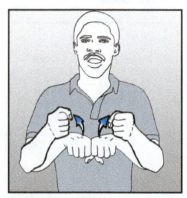

BREAK, snap

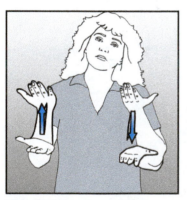

MAYBE, may, might

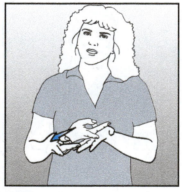

FAIL

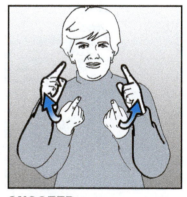

**SUCCEED,
success, successful**

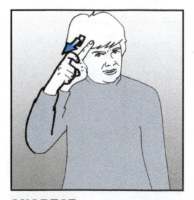

**SUSPECT,
suspicious, paranoid**

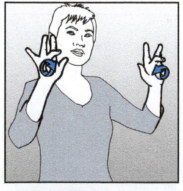

COMPUTER–1

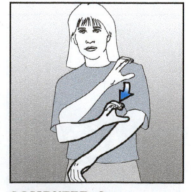

COMPUTER–2

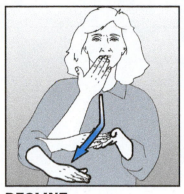

DECLINE

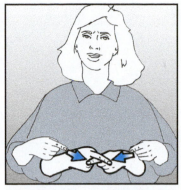

CONFLICT, contradiction

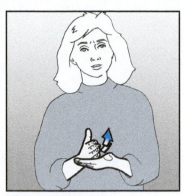

ALL-RIGHT, okay

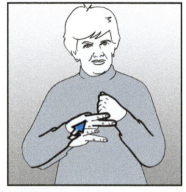

SAVE, preserve

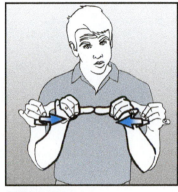

MEASURE

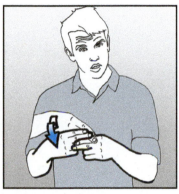

WEIGH, weight, pound

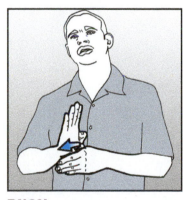

BUSY

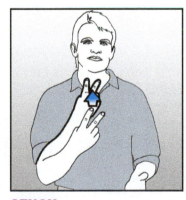

STUCK

12

UNIT 13

More Ways to Express Yourself

In this unit, you will learn more ways to express satisfaction or dissatisfaction, agreement or disagreement, and your concerns and feelings.

You will learn how to form conditional sentences.

You will also learn how to talk politely about death and dying.

SATISFACTION AND DISSATISFACTION

Pat: COME-ON, DOOR YOU-LOOK-AT-IT. NOT RIGHT IT. MUST AGAIN.

      whq   __whq___
Chris: WHY? WRONG?

Pat: SEE THERE DOOR CL:GG-AROUND-EDGE. LOUSY. NOT SATISFIED I.

      _____q_____
Chris: MUST I AGAIN?

        _____t_____
Pat: MUST. GOOD+ENOUGH, NOT ACCEPT I. MUST EXACT.

Key Structures

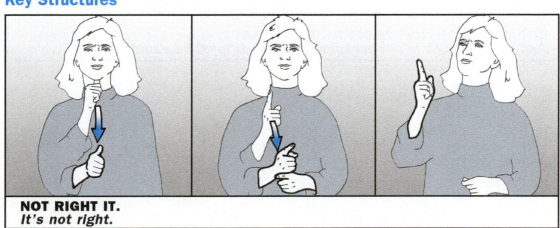

NOT RIGHT IT.
It's not right.

171

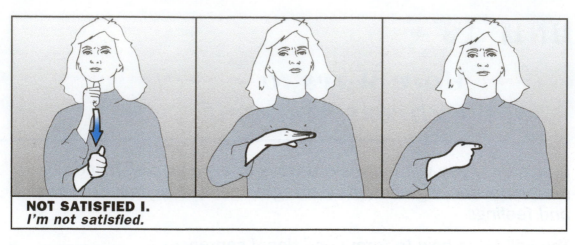

NOT SATISFIED I.
I'm not satisfied.

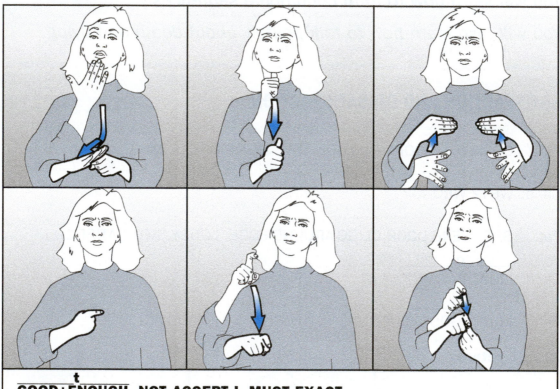

       t
GOOD+ENOUGH, NOT ACCEPT I. MUST EXACT.
Just good enough is not acceptable to me. It must be exact.

Note

Some ways to express satisfaction are:

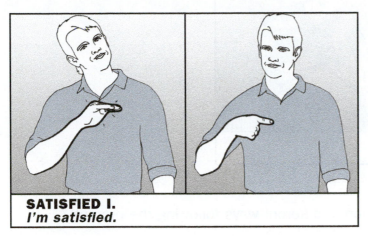

SATISFIED I.
I'm satisfied.

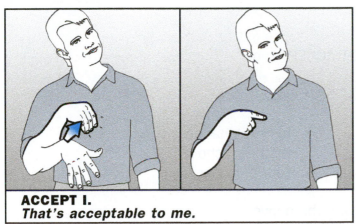

ACCEPT I.
That's acceptable to me.

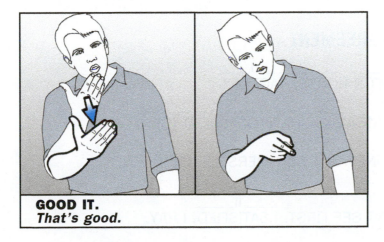

GOOD IT.
That's good.

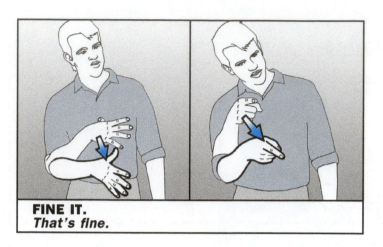

FINE IT.
That's fine.

Exercise 13A

a. Express your dissatisfaction in different ways following the prompt:

    Prompt: your work
             _____t_____
             YOUR WORK, NOT ACCEPT I. or
             _____t_____
             YOUR WORK, NOT SATISFIED I.

    1. the food   4. his explanation
    2. the car wash   5. the new school
    3. the bed   6. your behavior

b. Express your satisfaction with the above.

AGREEMENT AND DISAGREEMENT

           _____t_____ _____n_____
Lisa: THREE-OF-US LOOK-FOR HOUSE, I AGREE I.
           __whq__   _____q_____
Chris: #WHAT? I THINK SAME-AS-ME. HAVE DIFFERENT IDEA?

Lisa: MY IDEA TAKE-IT MONEY GIVE-HER. HERSELF DECIDE. NOT
        THREE-OF-US DECIDE.
                                            _____if_____
Chris: I DIFFERENT I. I WANT SEE FIRST. I SATISFIED, I PAY.

Lisa: I DISAGREE I.
           whq
Chris: #DO?

Key Structures

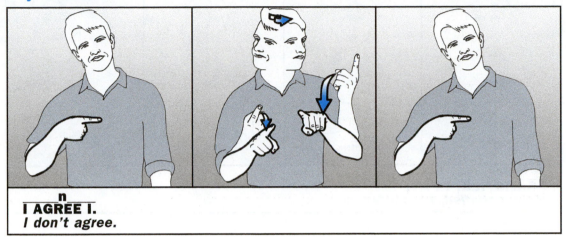

<u>I AGREE I.</u> ⁿ
I don't agree.

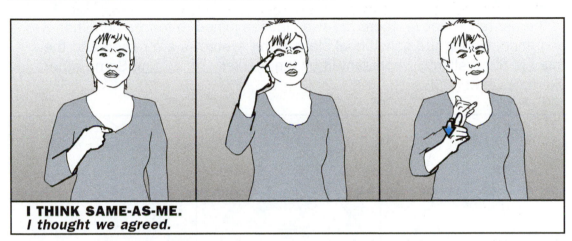

I THINK SAME-AS-ME.
I thought we agreed.

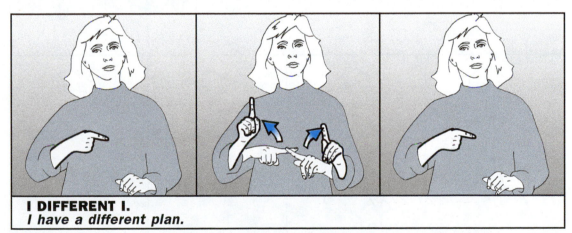

I DIFFERENT I.
I have a different plan.

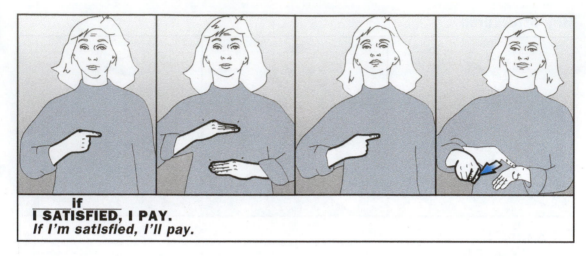

if
I SATISFIED, I PAY.
If I'm satisfied, I'll pay.

Grammar Note

In the sentence above, there are two clauses joined to form a conditional sentence. During the conditional clause, the eyebrows are raised and the head is tilted slightly (represented by the marker ____if____). Some other examples are:

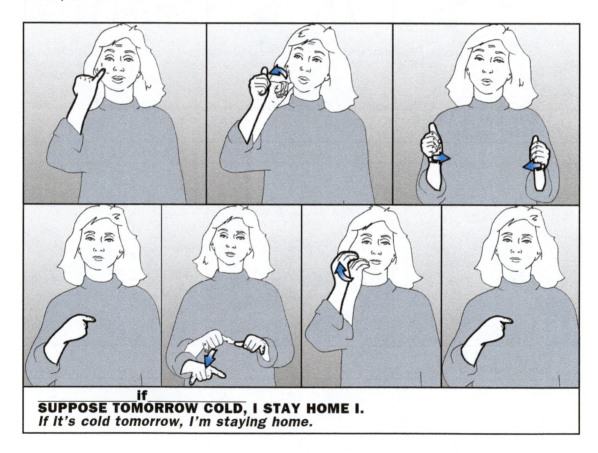

if
SUPPOSE TOMORROW COLD, I STAY HOME I.
If it's cold tomorrow, I'm staying home.

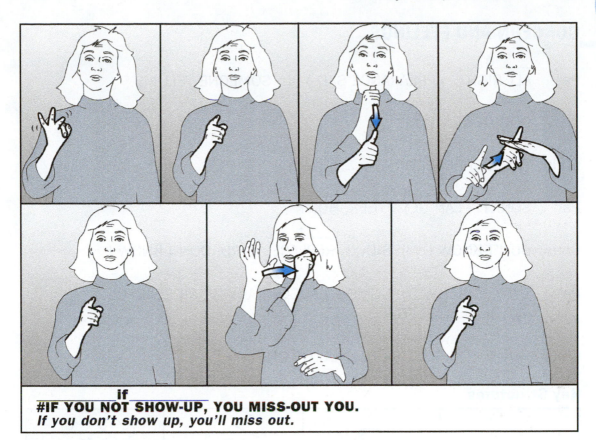

if
#IF YOU NOT SHOW-UP, YOU MISS-OUT YOU.
If you don't show up, you'll miss out.

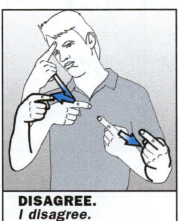

DISAGREE.
I disagree.

Exercise 13B

Indicate to your partner what you will do if the following happens.
Follow the prompt:

Prompt: his/her mother calls
_____ if _____
MOTHER TTY-TO-ME, I SUMMON-YOU.

1. it rains tomorrow
2. he/she is late
3. your car breaks down
4. you get the money
5. the letter doesn't arrive

6. the meeting is postponed
7. he/she doesn't arrive at 4:00
8. you buy food
9. you finish early
10. you see him

CONCERN AND FEELINGS

Pat: <u>_____q_____</u>
ALL-RIGHT? APPEARANCE SAD YOU. SOMEONE TELL-ME

<u>__q__</u>
DOG GONE. TRUE?

Chris: YES. DEPRESSED I.

Pat: <u>_____q_____</u>
SORRY. PLAN GET OTHER, HUH?

Chris: <u>____t____</u>
DON'T-KNOW I. MISS DOG. REPLACE, HARD. DON'T-KNOW I.

Pat: SYMPATHIZE-WITH. COME-ON ACCOMPANY-ME RIDE-BICYCLE,
MAYBE FEEL BETTER.

Chris: THANK-YOU. I ALL-RIGHT. YOU GO-ON.

Key Structures

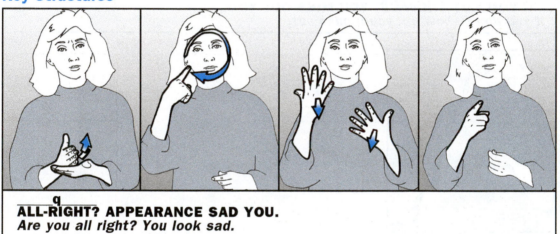

<u>_____q_____</u>
ALL-RIGHT? APPEARANCE SAD YOU.
Are you all right? You look sad.

Note

<u>_____q_____</u>
ALL-RIGHT? is used to ask about someone when you think something may be

<u>__whq__</u>
wrong or not going well. Two other ways to ask about someone are WRONG?,
which appears in previous units, and:

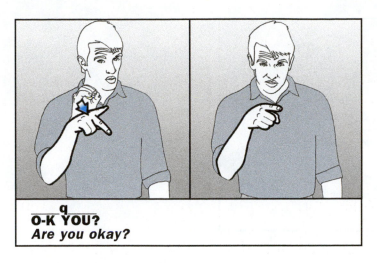

$\overline{\text{O-K}}^{\text{q}}\overline{\text{YOU?}}$
O-K YOU?
Are you okay?

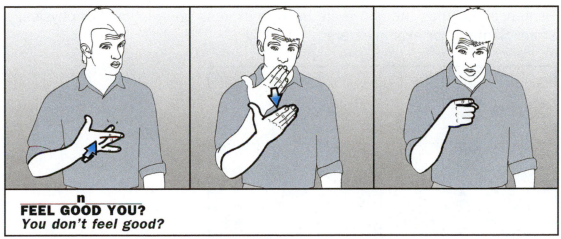

$\overline{\text{FEEL GOOD YOU?}}^{\text{n}}$
FEEL GOOD YOU?
You don't feel good?

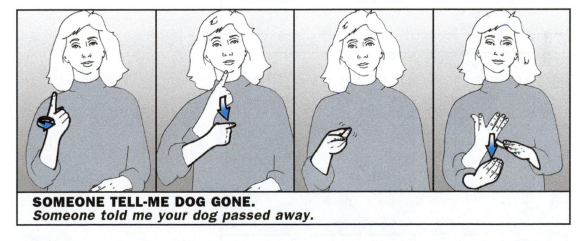

SOMEONE TELL-ME DOG GONE.
Someone told me your dog passed away.

Note

The use of GONE in the sentence above is a more polite and tactful way to mention the death of someone (or in the sentence above, a pet). DIE is acceptable when there is less concern about tactfulness.

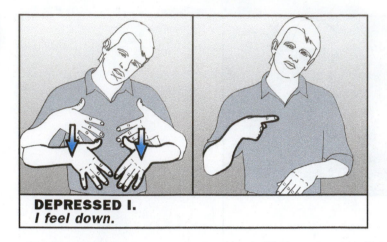

DEPRESSED I.
I feel down.

Grammar Note

Sentences such as the above are used to express an emotional or physical state. Some other examples are:

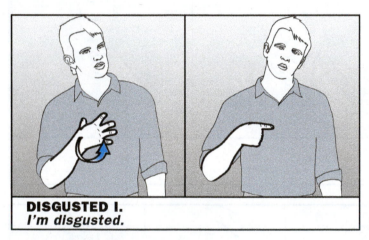

DISGUSTED I.
I'm disgusted.

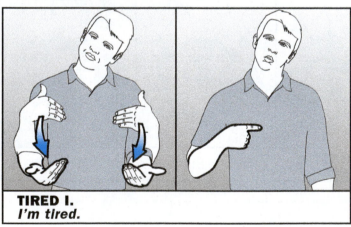

TIRED I.
I'm tired.

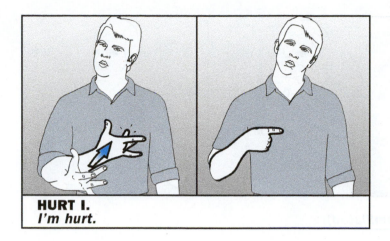

HURT I.
I'm hurt.

However, FEEL is usually used with emotional states rather than physical states. Note the meaning of the following examples:

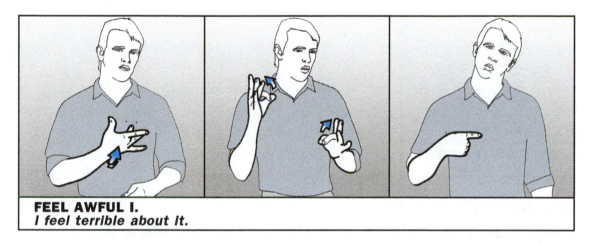

FEEL AWFUL I.
I feel terrible about it.

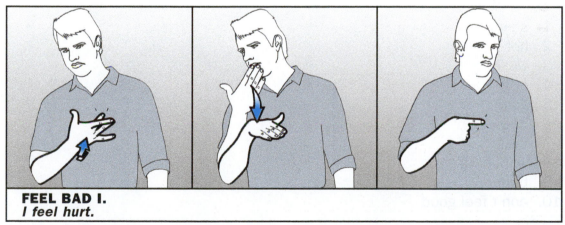

FEEL BAD I.
I feel hurt.

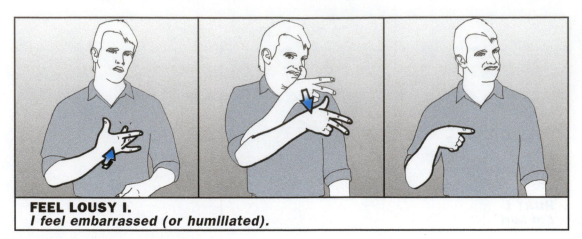

FEEL LOUSY I.
I feel embarrassed (or humiliated).

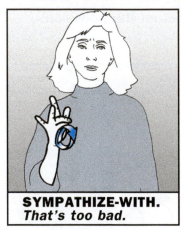

SYMPATHIZE-WITH.
That's too bad.

Exercise 13C

Describe your emotional or physical state to the student next to you.

1. sleepy
2. hot
3. weak
4. odd
5. good
6. bad
7. awful
8. wonderful
9. better
10. don't feel good

VOCABULARY

▶ Animals

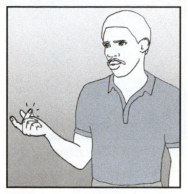

DOG

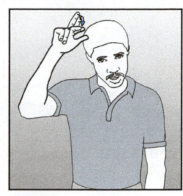

CAT, kitten

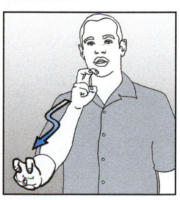

HORSE

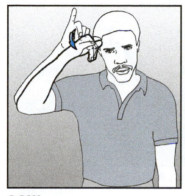

COW

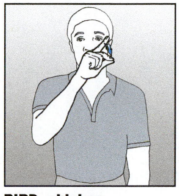

BIRD, chicken

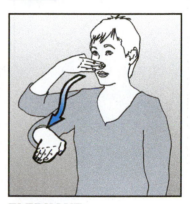

ELEPHANT

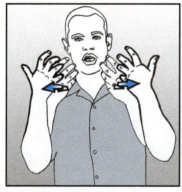

TIGER

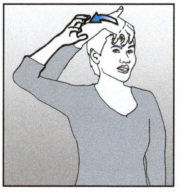

LION

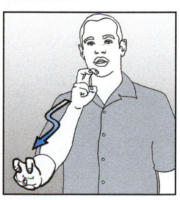

SNAKE

▶ Satisfaction

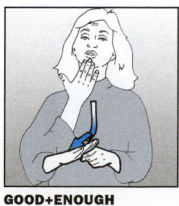

GOOD+ENOUGH

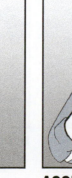

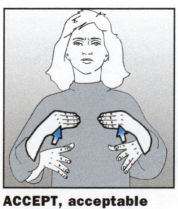

ACCEPT, acceptable

▶ Feelings

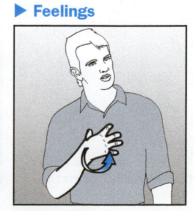

DISGUSTED

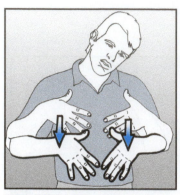

DEPRESSED, down

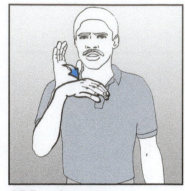

ODD, strange

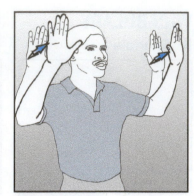

WONDERFUL, great

▶ **Other Vocabulary**

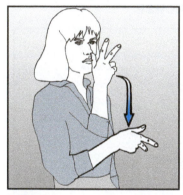

LOUSY

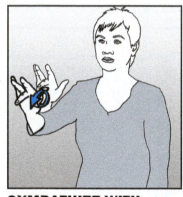

SYMPATHIZE-WITH, poor

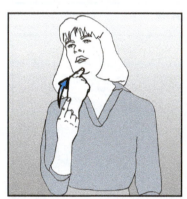

MISS

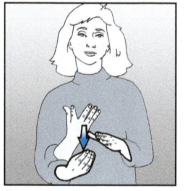

GONE

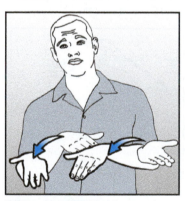

DIE, dead, died

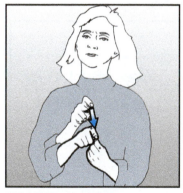

EXACT, precise

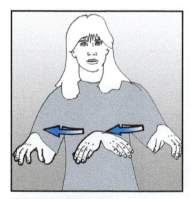

BEHAVIOR, do, act

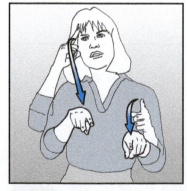

AGREE

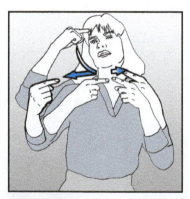

DISAGREE

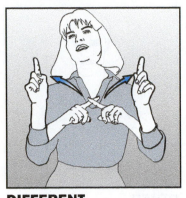

DIFFERENT

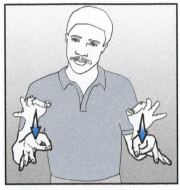

DECIDE, determine

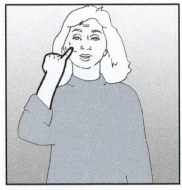

SUPPOSE, if

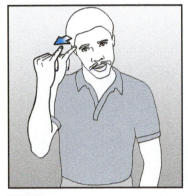

IDEA

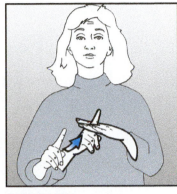

SHOW-UP, appear

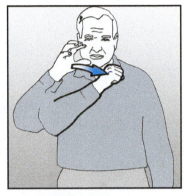

MISS-OUT, guess

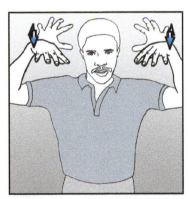

RAIN

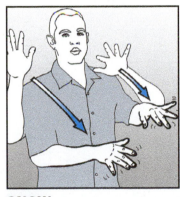

SNOW

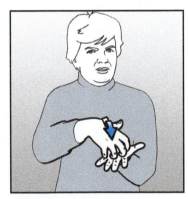

WEAK, vulnerable

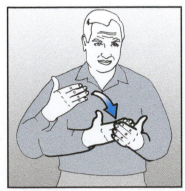

ARRIVE

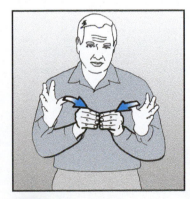

MEET,
Noun: MEETING

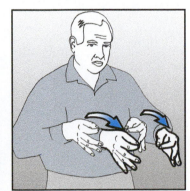

POSTPONE, put off

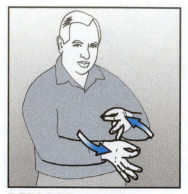 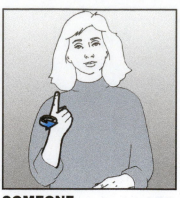 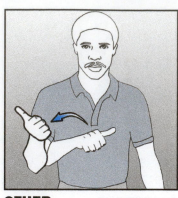

REPLACE, trade, exchange   **SOMEONE**   **OTHER**

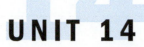

UNIT 14

Experiences and Current Activity

In this unit, you will learn how to talk about your experiences and what you are doing now. You will also learn how to ask what's happening and how to comment on someone's expertise or competence.

You will learn more classifiers that serve as quantifiers and you will learn about incorporating number into LAST-YEAR, NEXT-YEAR, LAST-WEEK, NEXT-WEEK, and NEXT-MONTH.

You will also learn different uses of FINISH and about conjunctions that join two clauses.

AN EVENT

Pat: I DECIDE GO-THERE SEE MOVIE. I ARRIVE. CAR CL:5̈5̈. I DRIVE-

AROUND 15 MINUTE. CAN'T PARK-CAR I. FINALLY CAR CL:3-BACK-OUT.

I CL:3-PULL-IN. I GO-THERE BUY TICKET, PEOPLE CL:44-LINE-OF-PEOPLE.

FINALLY I ENTER MOVIE, SIT. THINK-OF CAR LIGHT LIGHTS-ON,

      _____q_____
I TURN-LIGHTS-OFF? CAN'T REMEMBER I. I WATCH MOVIE FINISH I

RUN-THERE CAR. OF-COURSE BATTERY SHUT-DOWN.

Key Structures

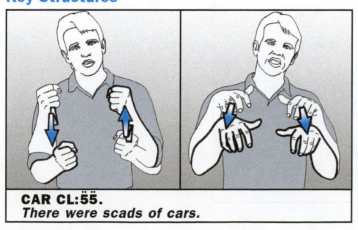

CAR CL:5̈5̈.
There were scads of cars.

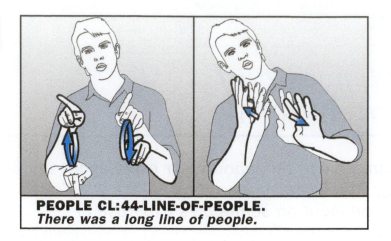

PEOPLE CL:44-LINE-OF-PEOPLE.
There was a long line of people.

Grammar Note

The classifiers in the two sentences above serve as quantifiers. They indicate the following:

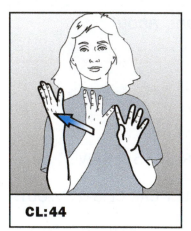

CL:44

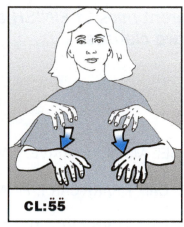

CL:55

A number of people, animals, objects in a line or row.

A large mass (people, animals, objects) over a large area.

Another classifier, CL:55⚌, is used to indicate a flowing mass (people, animals, etc.) as in:

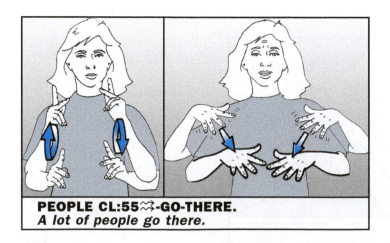

PEOPLE CL:55⚌-GO-THERE.
A lot of people go there.

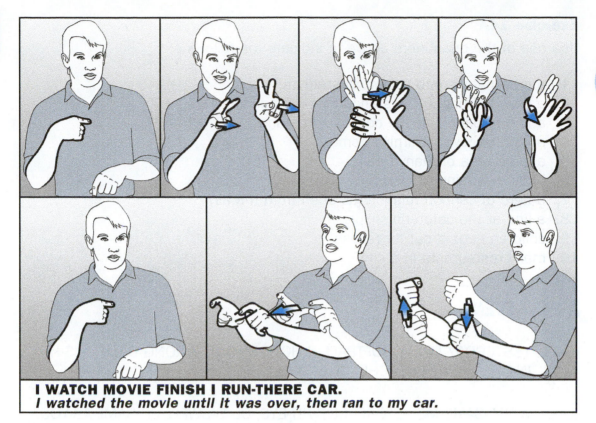

I WATCH MOVIE FINISH I RUN-THERE CAR.
I watched the movie until it was over, then ran to my car.

Grammar Note

FINISH can be used between clauses to indicate a sequence of events as in the sentence above and in the following:

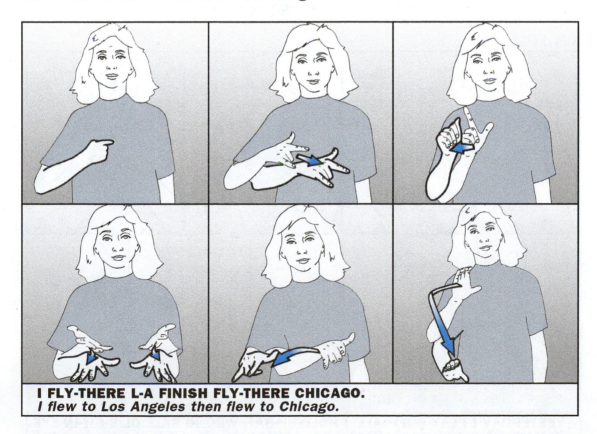

I FLY-THERE L-A FINISH FLY-THERE CHICAGO.
I flew to Los Angeles then flew to Chicago.

Exercise 14A

Use one of the quantifiers above to indicate the following:

1. a crowd going into a football stadium
2. a crowd sitting in the stands at a football game
3. a line of people at the concession stand
4. a herd of cows returning home
5. a large area of many trees
6. birds swarming to feed
7. a herd of caribou running (as seen from the air)
8. a line at the cafeteria
9. children getting out for recess
10. many restaurants in a city

A PAST EVENT

Chris: YESTERDAY I PLAY SOFTBALL. I HOLD-UP-BAT, WRONG BALL CL:S-HIT-IN-EYE. WOW! EYE-ACHE. CL:5̈-SWELL-UP.

Alex: WOW. SAME ME BEFORE. CL:B-HIT-EYE, CL-:5̈-SWELL-UP SAME-AS-YOU.

           __whq__
Chris: HAPPEN?

Alex: TWO-YEAR-AGO I DRIVE, WRONG CRASH CL:B-HIT-EYE.

Key Structures

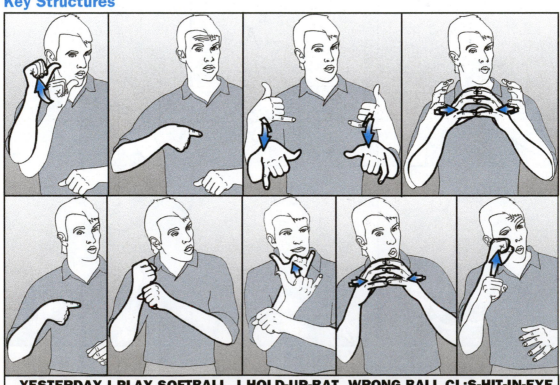

YESTERDAY I PLAY SOFTBALL. I HOLD-UP-BAT, WRONG BALL CL:S-HIT-IN-EYE.
Yesterday I was playing softball. I was batting and was hit in the eye by a ball.

14

Grammar Note

The previous sentence has two clauses joined by a conjunction, WRONG, which indicates an unexpected, but not necessarily unpleasant, event. Other conjunctions that indicate unexpected events are:

HAPPEN, for unexpected events;
FIND, for unexpected discoveries;
FRUSTRATED, for unexpected obstacles;
and HIT, for unexpectedly lucking out.

Some examples are:

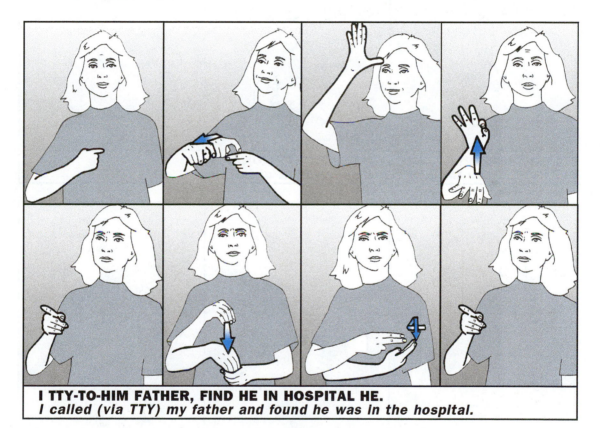

I TTY-TO-HIM FATHER, FIND HE IN HOSPITAL HE.
I called (via TTY) my father and found he was in the hospital.

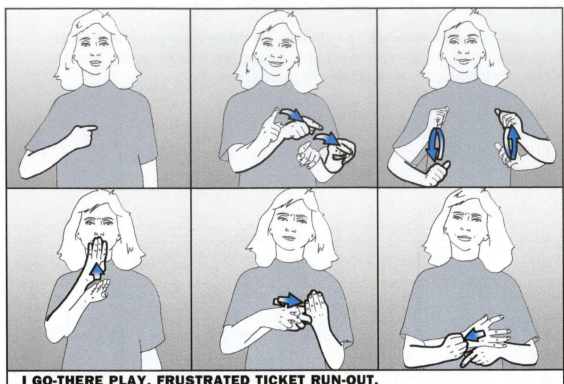

I GO-THERE PLAY, FRUSTRATED TICKET RUN-OUT.
I went to see the play but they were out of tickets.

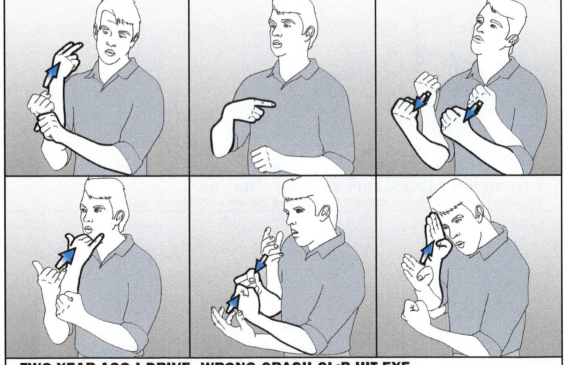

TWO-YEAR-AGO I DRIVE, WRONG CRASH CL:B-HIT-EYE.
Two years ago while I was driving, I had an accident and was hit in the eye.

Grammar Note

As in the previous sentence, the numbers one to five can be incorporated into LAST-YEAR or NEXT-YEAR to indicate how many years ago or how many years from now. Numbers above five are not incorporated but are used with YEAR. Some examples are:

14

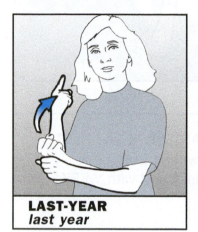

LAST-YEAR
last year

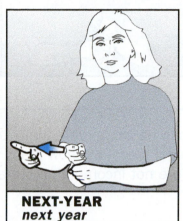

NEXT-YEAR
next year

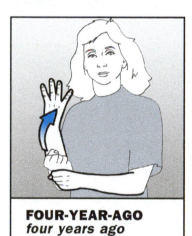

FOUR-YEAR-AGO
four years ago

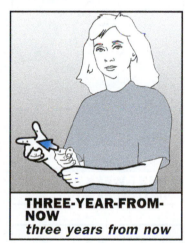

THREE-YEAR-FROM-NOW
three years from now

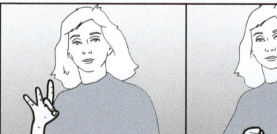
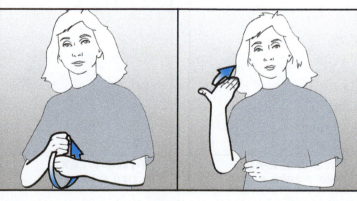

8 YEAR PAST
8 years ago

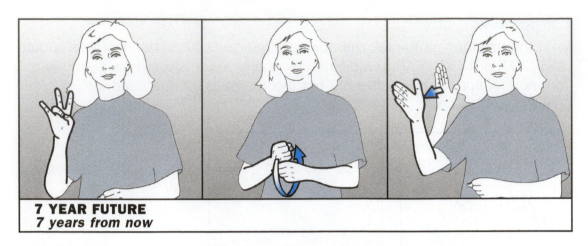

7 YEAR FUTURE
7 years from now

The numbers one to nine can be incorporated into LAST-WEEK and NEXT-WEEK to show how many weeks ago and how many weeks from now. Numbers higher than nine are not incorporated but are used with WEEK. Some examples are:

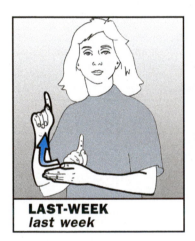

LAST-WEEK
last week

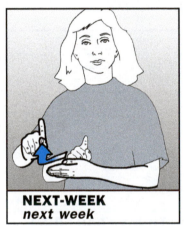

NEXT-WEEK
next week

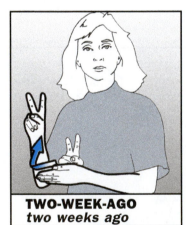

TWO-WEEK-AGO
two weeks ago

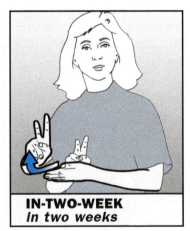

IN-TWO-WEEK
In two weeks

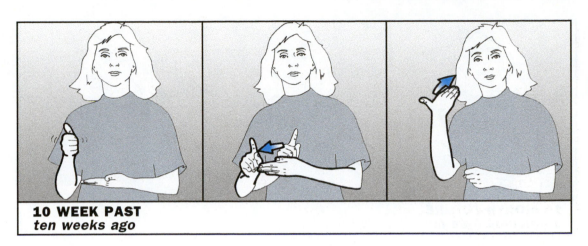

10 WEEK PAST
ten weeks ago

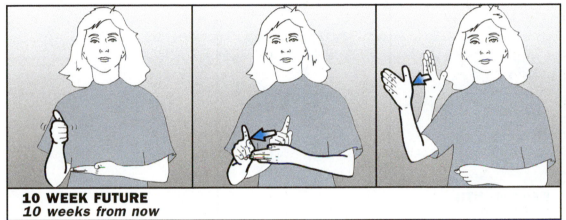

10 WEEK FUTURE
10 weeks from now

NEXT-MONTH can incorporate the numbers one to nine to show how many months from now. However, there is no number incorporation showing how many months in the past. Some examples are:

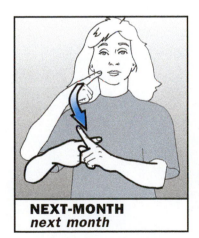

NEXT-MONTH
next month

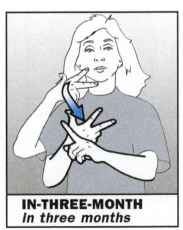

IN-THREE-MONTH
In three months

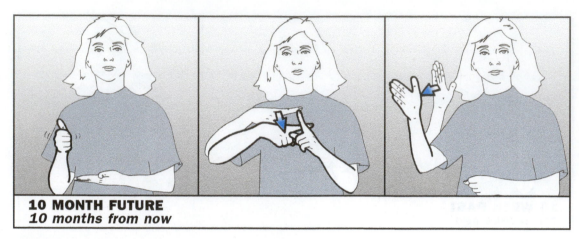

10 MONTH FUTURE
10 months from now

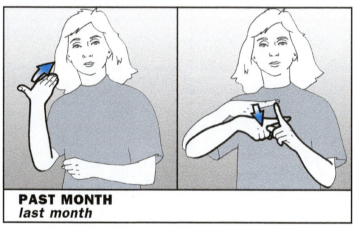

PAST MONTH
last month

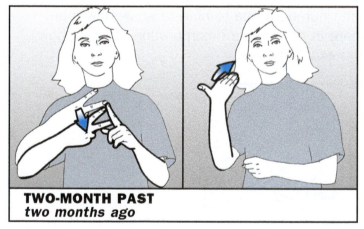

TWO-MONTH PAST
two months ago

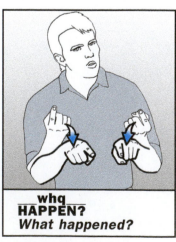

whq
HAPPEN?
What happened?

Grammar Note

Other ways to ask what happened or what's happening are:

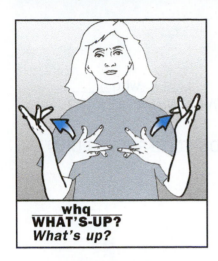

___whq___
WHAT'S-UP?
What's up?

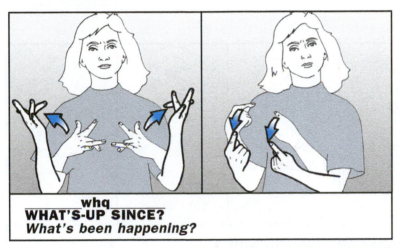

___whq___
WHAT'S-UP SINCE?
What's been happening?

Exercise 14B

a. Use the five conjunctions to tell about five unexpected events that happened to you.

b. Indicate how many years ago and complete the sentence.
Follow the prompt.

Prompt: 7

7 YEAR PAST I _____.

1. 3   6. 5
2. 19   7. 4
3. 8   8. 2
4. 21   9. 10
5. 1   10. 6

CURRENT ACTIVITY

         _____whq_____

Lisa: WHAT'S-UP?

        _____t_____

Chris: CABINET OLD I TAKE-OUT, PUT-IN NEW.

     _____t_____   _____whq_____

Lisa: YOU GOOD-AT DO-WOODWORK, DON'T-KNOW I. WHERE LEARN?

Chris: SCHOOL-FOR-DEAF THERE. NOW I MAKE DOOR CL:B-ROUND-EDGE-ON-CL:B.

Lisa: WOW. SKILL YOU.

      _____if_____

Chris: HAVE MACHINE, EASY.

Key Structures

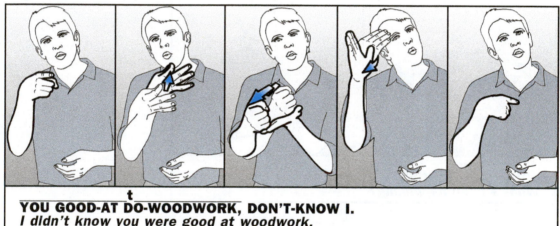

                     t
YOU GOOD-AT DO-WOODWORK, DON'T-KNOW I.
I didn't know you were good at woodwork.

Grammar Note

GOOD-AT, as in the previous sentence, is one of several ways to comment on one's competence or expertise. Some examples are:

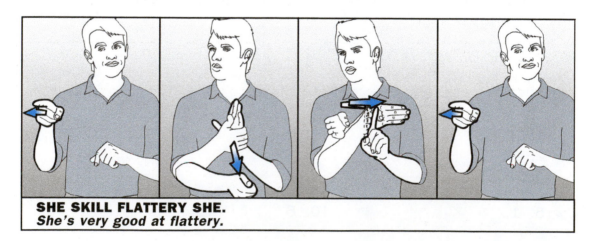

SHE SKILL FLATTERY SHE.
She's very good at flattery.

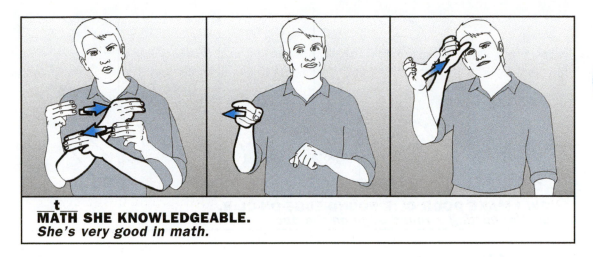

<u>t</u>
MATH SHE KNOWLEDGEABLE.
She's very good in math.

Some ways to comment on one's lack of competence or expertise are:

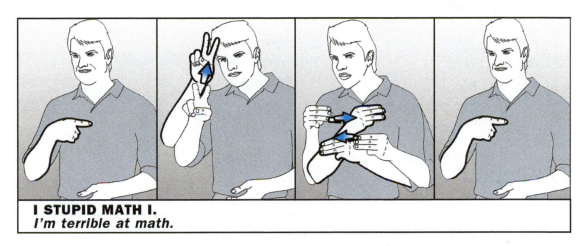

I STUPID MATH I.
I'm terrible at math.

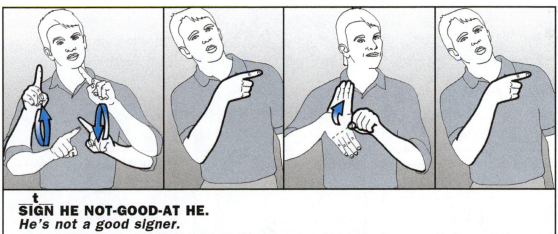

<u>t</u>
SIGN HE NOT-GOOD-AT HE.
He's not a good signer.

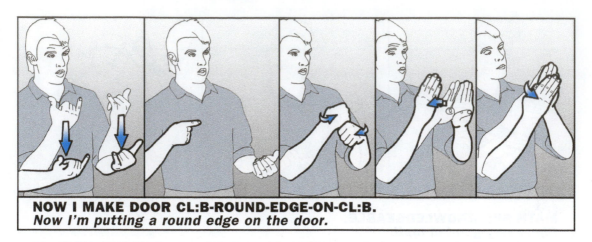

NOW I MAKE DOOR CL:B-ROUND-EDGE-ON-CL:B.
Now I'm putting a round edge on the door.

Exercise 14C

Comment on your competence or expertise in the following:

1. history
2. art
3. swimming
4. softball
5. basketball

6. cooking
7. typing
8. dancing
9. driving
10. computers

VOCABULARY

▶ **Sports**

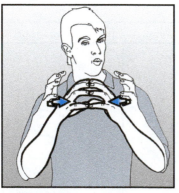

SOFTBALL

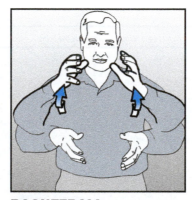

BASKETBALL

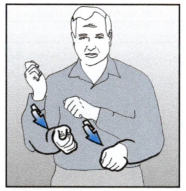

BASEBALL

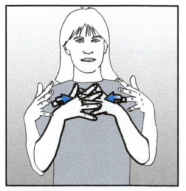

FOOTBALL

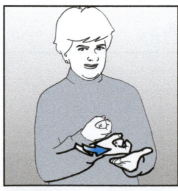

HOCKEY

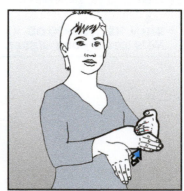

SOCCER

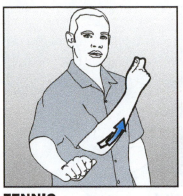

TENNIS

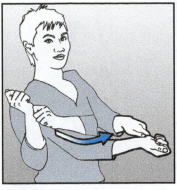

GOLF

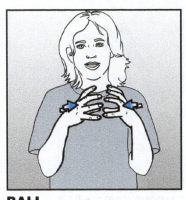

BALL

▶ **Conjunctions**

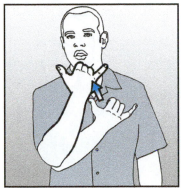
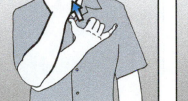

WRONG

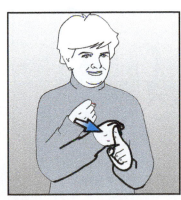

HAPPEN, when

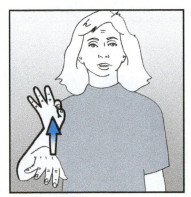

FIND, discover

▶ **Expressing
Competence or
Incompetence**

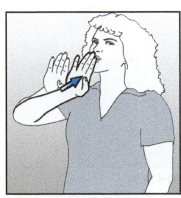
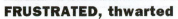

FRUSTRATED, thwarted

HIT

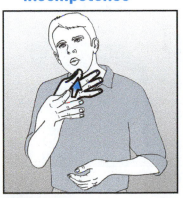

GOOD-AT

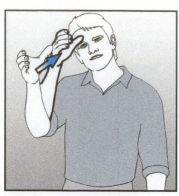

KNOWLEDGEABLE, genius

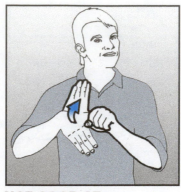

NOT-GOOD-AT, incompetent, inept

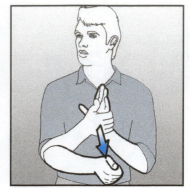

SKILL, expert, competent

▶ **Noun-Verb Pairs**

▶ **Places**

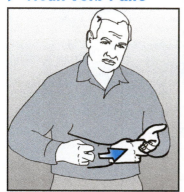

GIVE-TICKET, Noun: TICKET

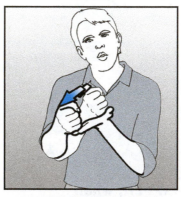

DO-WOODWORK, Noun: CARPENTER, CARPENTRY

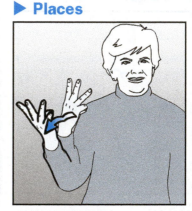

WASHINGTON

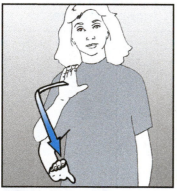

CHICAGO

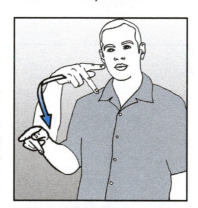

PHILADELPHIA

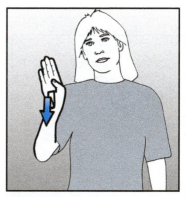

BOSTON

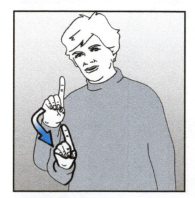

DETROIT

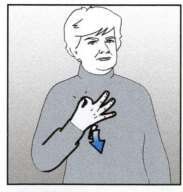

PITTSBURGH

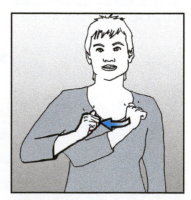

ATLANTA

14

▶ **Subjects**

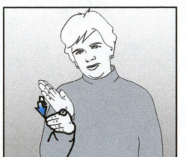

BALTIMORE

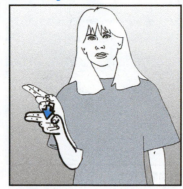

HISTORY

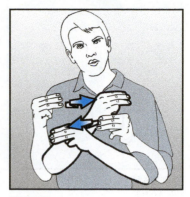

MATH

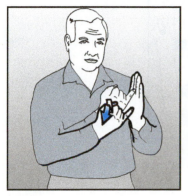

ART

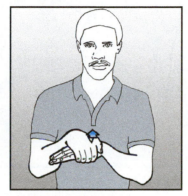

ENGLISH, England, British

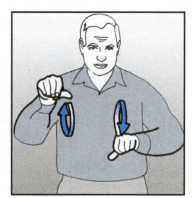

SCIENCE

▶ **Other Vocabulary**

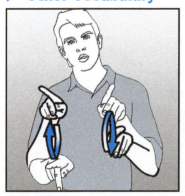

PEOPLE

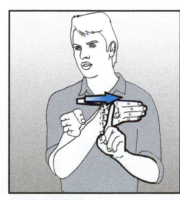

FLATTERY

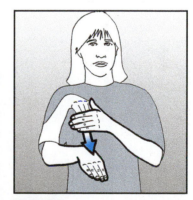

ENTER

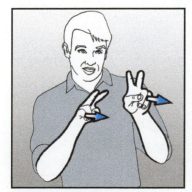

WATCH, look at

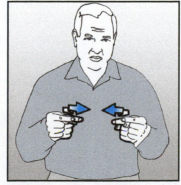

HURT, pain, injury

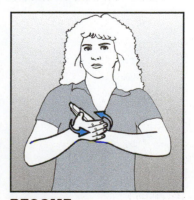

BECOME

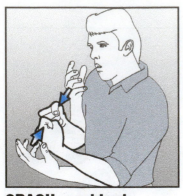

CRASH, accident

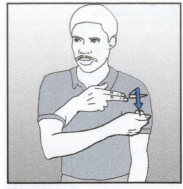

HOSPITAL

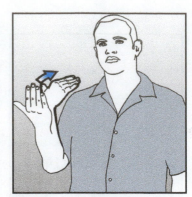

PAST, before, ago

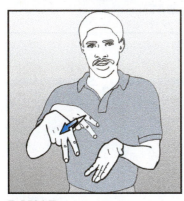

DANCE

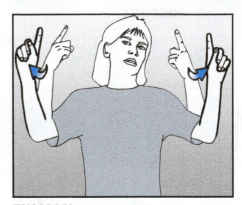

FINALLY

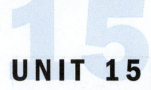

UNIT 15

Future Plans and Obligations

15

In this unit, you will talk about plans and future obligations.

You will learn about verb pairs such as GET-IN and GET-OUT, and GET-ON and GET-OFF.

And in culture notes, you will learn about movie and TV captioning, as well as about Deaf clubs and their history.

GENERAL FUTURE PLANS

```
                   t
       _____t_____
Lisa:  GRADUATE H-S FINISH, GO-THERE COLLEGE I.
```

Chris: DON'T-WANT COLLEGE I.

```
       _____t_____ _whq_
Lisa:  GRADUATE, #DO?
```

Chris: WANT #JOB EASY, ORDINARY. PRESSURE, DON'T-WANT I.

```
       _____q_____
Lisa:  MARRY, CHILDREN WILL YOU?
```

Chris: DON'T-KNOW I. I THINK-ABOUT I.

Key Structures

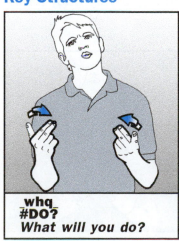

whq
#DO?
What will you do?

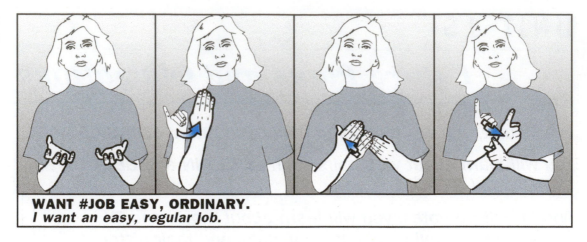

WANT #JOB EASY, ORDINARY.
I want an easy, regular job.

Note

ORDINARY in the above sentence is used to express that something is the regular, expected, or usual.

NOTHING-TO-IT is another way to express that something is not unusual as in:

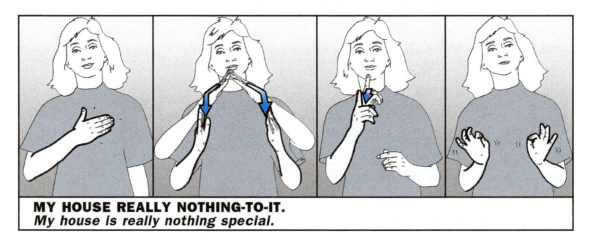

MY HOUSE REALLY NOTHING-TO-IT.
My house is really nothing special.

NOTHING-TO-IT can also be used to express that something is very easy as in the following:

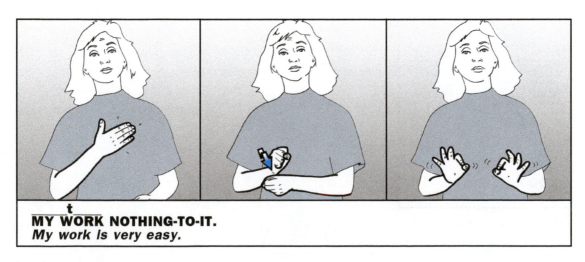

                                              t
MY WORK NOTHING-TO-IT.
My work is very easy.

Or, more negatively, unimportant, or without substance:

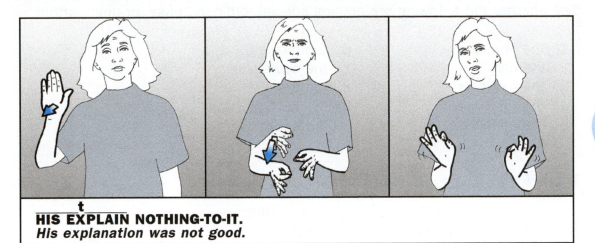

$\overline{\text{HIS EXP}}$$\overset{\text{t}}{\overline{\text{LAIN}}}$ NOTHING-TO-IT.
His explanation was not good.

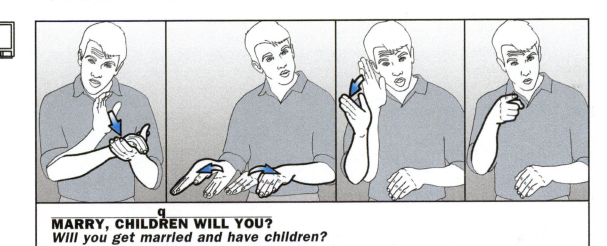

$\overline{\text{MARRY, CHIL}}$$\overset{\text{q}}{\overline{\text{DREN}}}$ WILL YOU?
Will you get married and have children?

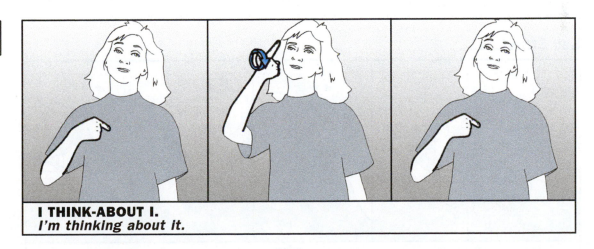

I THINK-ABOUT I.
I'm thinking about it.

Exercise 15A

Tell whether the following are nothing special, ordinary, easy, or unimportant.

1. the house
2. the car
3. the furniture
4. the food
5. the homework

6. the movie
7. the course
8. the test
9. the work
10. the book

TIME AND PLACE TO MEET

<pre>
            _____t_____   _whq_
Alex: NEXT-WEEK I-MEET-YOU, I PICK-UP TIME?

            _____q_____
Pat: GO-THERE L-A YOU MEAN?

          whq
Alex: YES. TIME?

                         _q_
Pat: TIME-8, MORNING. O-K?

Alex: FINE. I I-MEET-YOU YOUR HOUSE, YOU GET-IN MY CAR.

Pat: O-K. I WAIT OUTSIDE. I STAND FRONT.

            _____if_____
Alex: SUPPOSE TRAFFIC BAD, MAYBE I LATE. BE-PATIENT WAIT.
       I SHOW-UP WILL.
</pre>

Key Structures

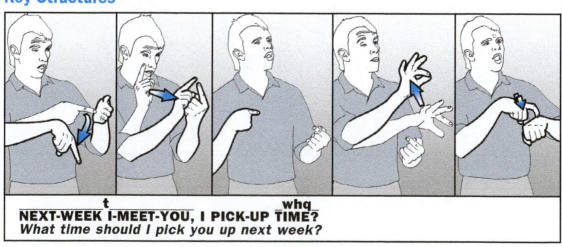

_____t_____   _whq_
NEXT-WEEK I-MEET-YOU, I PICK-UP TIME?
What time should I pick you up next week?

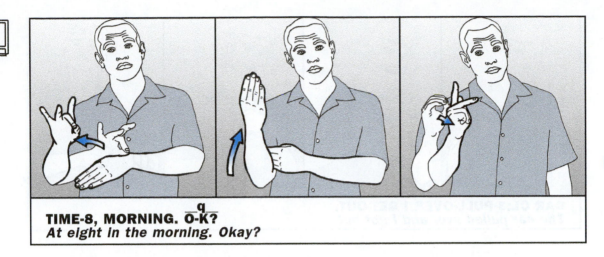

TIME-8, MORNING. O-K?
At eight in the morning. Okay?

15

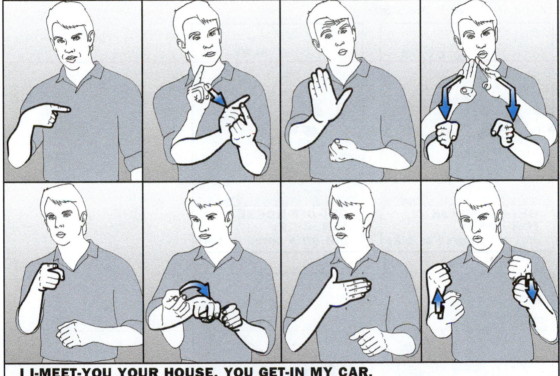

I I-MEET-YOU YOUR HOUSE, YOU GET-IN MY CAR.
I'll meet you at your house and you can join me in my car.

Grammar Note

GET-IN and GET-OUT is a verb pair to indicate getting in and out of vehicles including cars, trains, and planes. GET-OUT is shown in the following sentence:

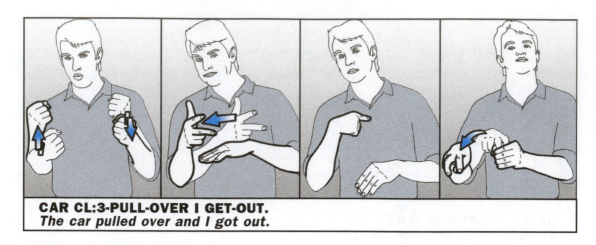

CAR CL:3-PULL-OVER I GET-OUT.
The car pulled over and I got out.

Some other verb pairs are:

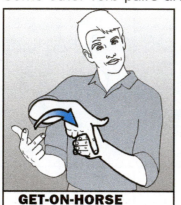

GET-ON-HORSE (OR -BIKE)
get on a horse or bike

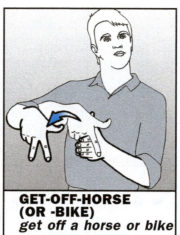

GET-OFF-HORSE (OR -BIKE)
get off a horse or bike

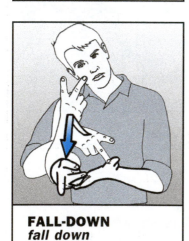

FALL-DOWN
fall down

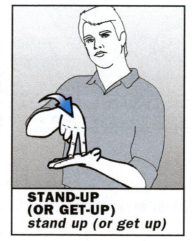

STAND-UP (OR GET-UP)
stand up (or get up)

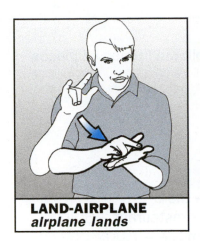

LAND-AIRPLANE
airplane lands

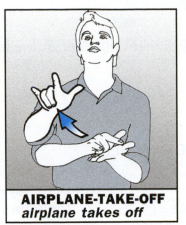

AIRPLANE-TAKE-OFF
airplane takes off

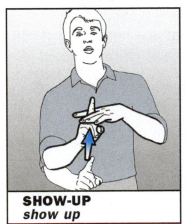

SHOW-UP
show up

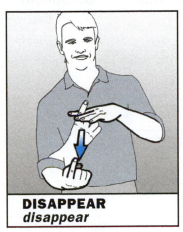

DISAPPEAR
disappear

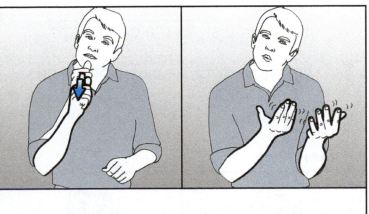

YOU BE-PATIENT WAIT.
Be patient and wait.

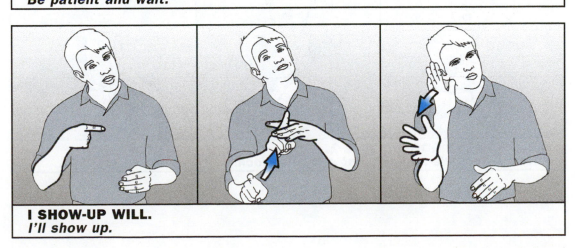

I SHOW-UP WILL.
I'll show up.

15

Exercise 15B

Tell your partner that you will meet him/her at the following times or places. Follow the prompt:

Prompt: next week - here

NEXT-WEEK I-MEET-YOU HERE.

1. Tuesday – 4:00
2. next month – my house
3. next week – Monday – 10:00
4. Fridays – 3:00
5. Wednesday – here
6. Saturday – there
7. tomorrow – restaurant – 6:30
8. Sunday – movie – 7:00
9. in two weeks – Washington
10. in three months – here

FUTURE OBLIGATIONS

```
                    _____q_____
Chris: TWO-OF-US GO-THERE SWIM?

Alex:  CAN'T I. APPOINTMENT DOCTOR TIME-2.

                         _____q_____
Chris: OH-I-SEE. CAN TOMORROW NIGHT COME-HERE MY HOUSE

       _____
       CL:L-PUT-IN-DISK WATCH CAPTIONED?

Alex:  NO. STUCK DUTY, WORK THERE #CLUB.

Chris: WOW. BUSY YOU. SHOULD I APPOINTMENT TWO-MONTH PAST.
```

Key Structures

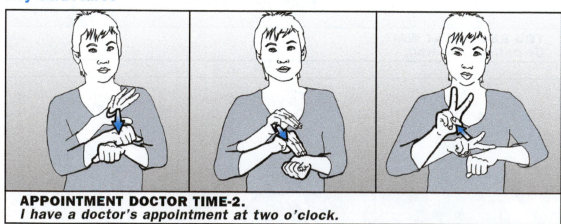

APPOINTMENT DOCTOR TIME-2.
I have a doctor's appointment at two o'clock.

Grammar Note

Some other ways to indicate an obligation are:

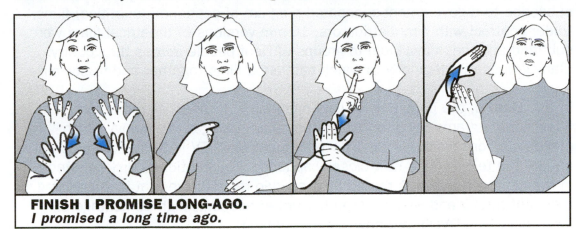

FINISH I PROMISE LONG-AGO.
I promised a long time ago.

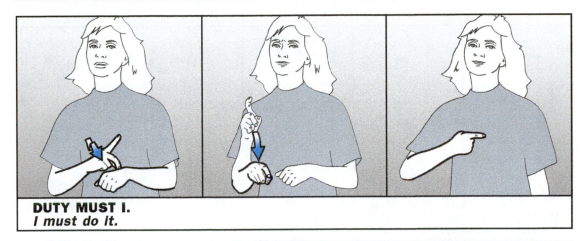

DUTY MUST I.
I must do it.

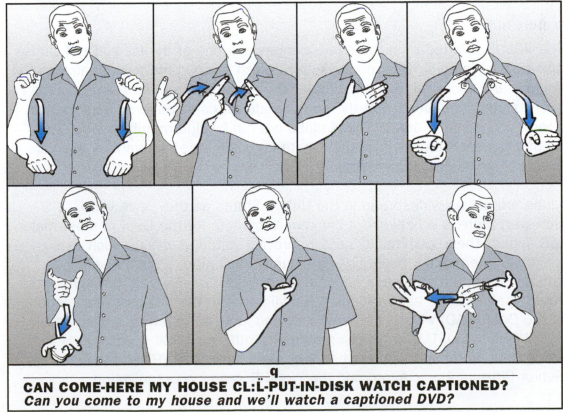

CAN COME-HERE MY HOUSE CL:L̈-PUT-IN-DISK WATCH CAPTIONED?
Can you come to my house and we'll watch a captioned DVD?

15

Culture Note

Beginning in the 1950's, and to some extent today, Deaf people could subscribe to a government-sponsored program of captioned (subtitled) films. Under contract with film distributors, 16-mm versions of theatrical films were subtitled and made available to groups of Deaf people across the country. Many groups met regularly to watch captioned films together and to socialize.

In the 1980's, the popularity of captioned films declined as more and more television programs became closed-captioned. Using a technology which makes captions visible when a decoder built into a TV is turned on, much of prime time television is now closed-captioned. The captioned disk referred to in the sentence above is rented from a video rental store. Pat is suggesting they rent a DVD and watch it together at her house. A high percentage of videotapes and DVD's are now close-captioned.

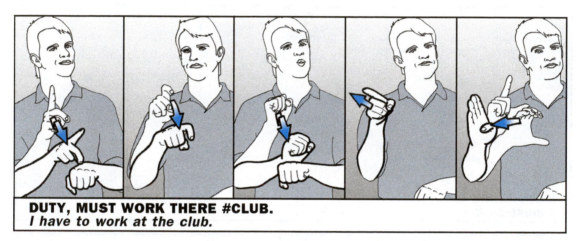

DUTY, MUST WORK THERE #CLUB.
I have to work at the club.

Culture Note

The #CLUB referred to in the above sentence is one of the local "Deaf clubs," still existing in some Deaf communities, which at one time were central to the cultural and social life of Deaf people. These clubs range from sports clubs to social clubs sometimes with their own buildings, complete with bars, dance floors, and meeting areas. These clubs are run by club members who serve as officers, staff the bars, or participate on committees for various special events. Terry is one such member.

Clubs are not as widespread in the United States as they once were. However, there is a network of community centers for the Deaf in most major U.S. cities. These community centers provide various services such as sign language interpreting, advocacy, community education, and counseling. In addition there are state and national associations of the Deaf throughout the country. Most state associations are affiliated with the National Association of the Deaf (NAD) which is an advocacy and lobbying organization located near Washington, D.C. In addition there are other national associations with many Deaf members such as the Black Deaf Advocates (BDA), the Deaf Senior Citizens Association, and the World Recreation Organization.

Exercise 15C

In response to a request to go shopping tomorrow, apologize and give the following prior commitments:

1. You must visit your grandfather.
2. You have reservations to fly to Chicago.
3. You have an appointment to see a lawyer.
4. You have to go to court.
5. You are committed to meet a friend.
6. You must be with your family.
7. You must work at the club.
8. You must see your doctor.
9. You must wash your car.
10. You must drive to Philadelphia.

VOCABULARY

▶ Verb Pairs

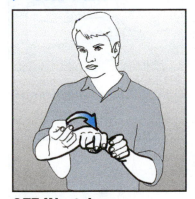

GET-IN, get on

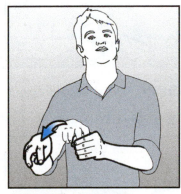

GET-OUT, get off

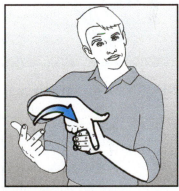

GET-ON, mount

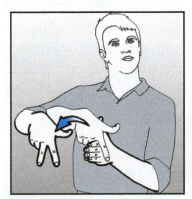

GET-OFF, dismount

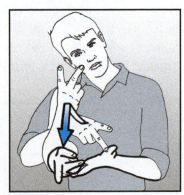

FALL-DOWN

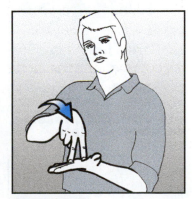

STAND-UP

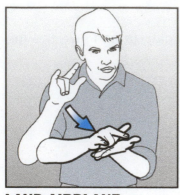

LAND-AIRPLANE

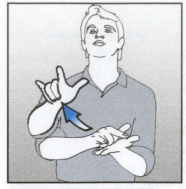

AIRPLANE-TAKE-OFF

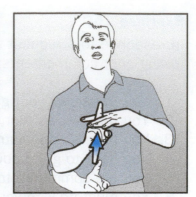

SHOW-UP, appear

▶ **Commitment**

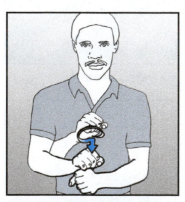

DISAPPEAR, vanish

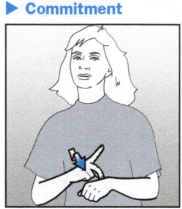

DUTY, obligation

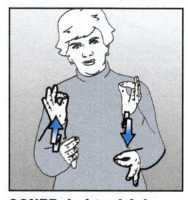

PROMISE, commitment

▶ **Legal Terms**

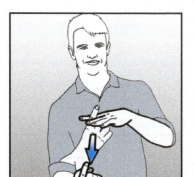

APPOINTMENT, reserve, reservation, date

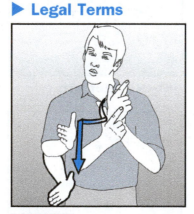

LAWYER

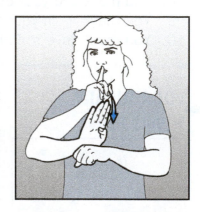

COURT, judge, trial

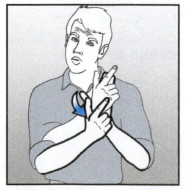

LAW, legal

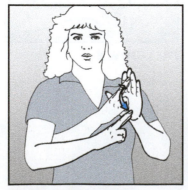

RULE, regulation

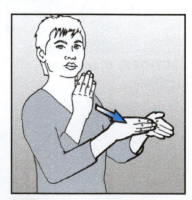

SUE

▶ Position

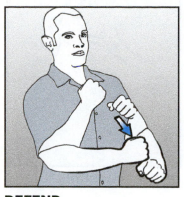

DEFEND

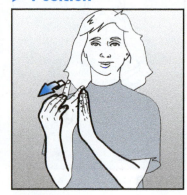

OUTSIDE

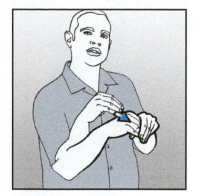

INSIDE, within

15

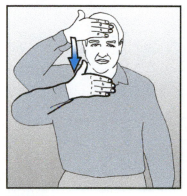

FRONT

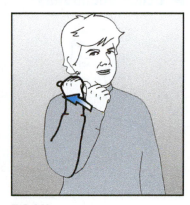

BACK

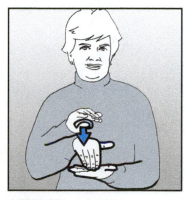

CENTER, middle

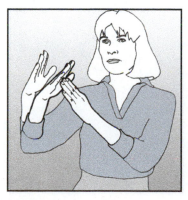

TOP

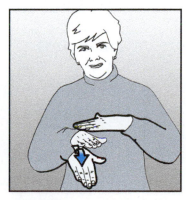

BOTTOM

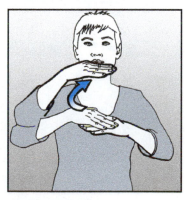

ABOVE, over

▶ Eating Out

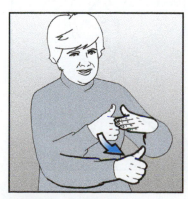

UNDER, beneath

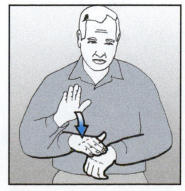

ON

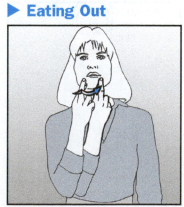

RESTAURANT

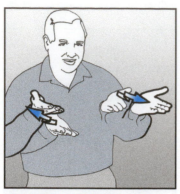

WAITER/WAITRESS

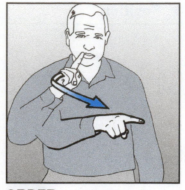

ORDER

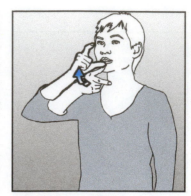

DRINK, cocktail

▶ **Other Vocabulary**

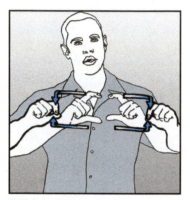

BILL, check

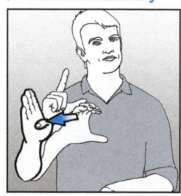

#CLUB

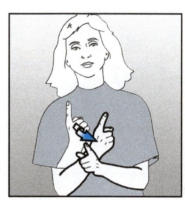

ORDINARY

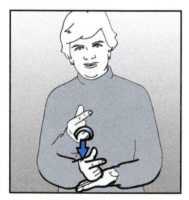

GRADUATE

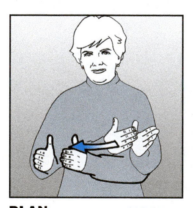

PLAN

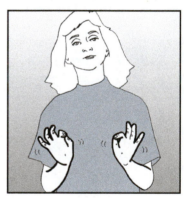

NOTHING-TO-IT

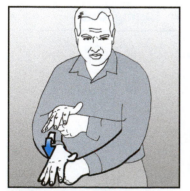

PRESSURE, stress

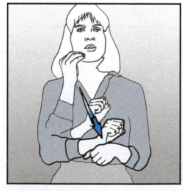

HOME+WORK

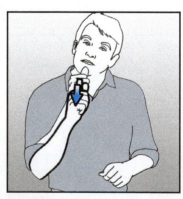

BE-PATIENT

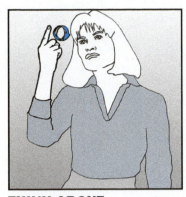

THINK-ABOUT

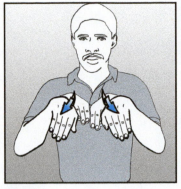

SWIM

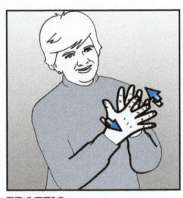

TRAFFIC

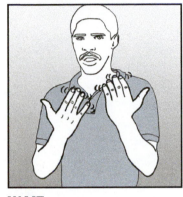

WAIT

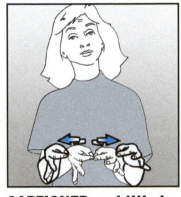

CAPTIONED, subtitled

15

UNIT 16

Directions and Instructions

In this unit, you will learn how to give directions and instructions. You will learn how to use the body as well as some classifiers to show locational relationships.

You will learn about some commonly used fingerspelled abbreviations and about making apostrophes in fingerspelling names. You will learn about showing the possessive without using an apostrophe.

You will also learn a new instrument classifier.

16

DIRECTIONS

<pre>   ____q____
Pat: EXCUSE-ME. HAVE D-S NEAR?
</pre>

Alex: YES. YOU OUT, LEFT. DRIVE INTERSECTION++, LEFT. STRAIGHT TWO INTERSECTION, INTERSECTION, THERE CORNER.

<pre>   ___whq___
Pat: HOW I OUT?
</pre>

<pre>   _____q_____
Alex: OH-I-SEE. BEFORE HERE NEVER YOU?
</pre>

Pat: NEVER I.

Alex: O-K. THERE ELEVATOR DOWN FIRST FLOOR, RIGHT, THERE OUT.

Key Structures

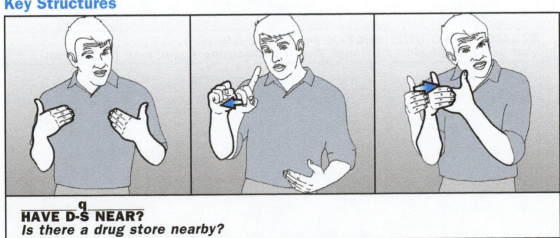

<pre>   q
HAVE D-S NEAR?
</pre>
Is there a drug store nearby?

221

Note

D-S for drug store, H-S for high school, and P-O for post office are commonly used fingerspelled abbreviations.

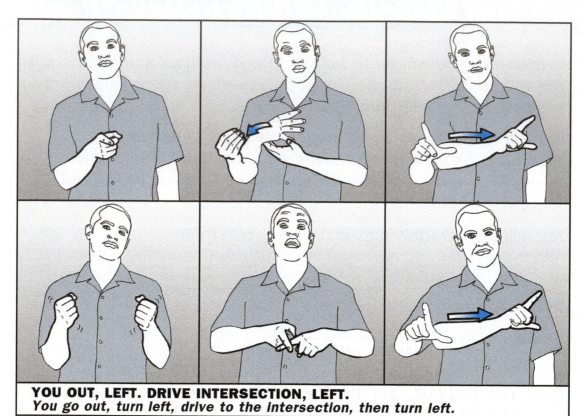

YOU OUT, LEFT. DRIVE INTERSECTION, LEFT.
You go out, turn left, drive to the intersection, then turn left.

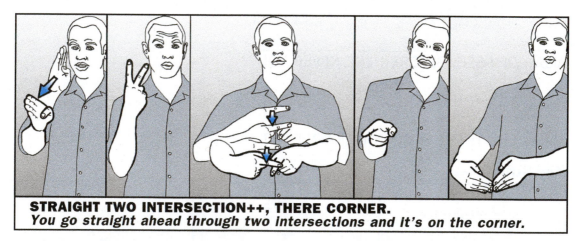

STRAIGHT TWO INTERSECTION++, THERE CORNER.
You go straight ahead through two intersections and it's on the corner.

Grammar Note

When giving directions, sometimes the position of the hands and the body are used to show change in direction.

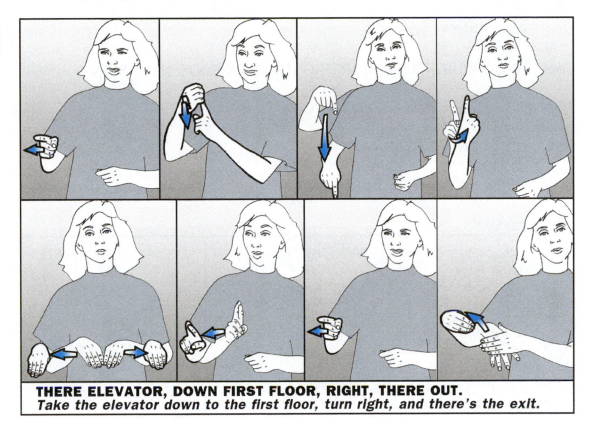

THERE ELEVATOR, DOWN FIRST FLOOR, RIGHT, THERE OUT.
Take the elevator down to the first floor, turn right, and there's the exit.

16

Exercise 16A

Give directions for your partner to get to the following:

1. the drugstore
2. the post office
3. the high school
4. the food store
5. the police station
6. the hospital
7. the restaurant
8. the bookstore
9. the cafeteria
10. the library

DESCRIPTIONS OF PLACES

                                        q
Chris: WANT TWO-OF-US GO-AWAY RESTAURANT J-O-S-E-apostrophe-S?

Lisa: DON'T-KNOW WHERE I.

Chris: KNOW WHITE CL:BB-STOREFRONT, GREEN ROOF. HAVE SIGN
                              q
       J-O-S-E-apostrophe-S. KNOW YOU?
                 whq
Lisa: DON'T-KNOW. NEAR WHAT?

Chris: TEMPLE CL:A> RESTAURANT CL:A>.

Key Structures

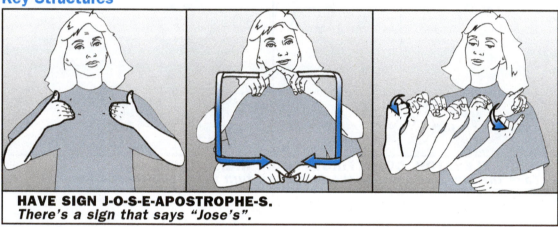

HAVE SIGN J-O-S-E-APOSTROPHE-S.
There's a sign that says "Jose's".

Note

When it is necessary to give an exact fingerspelled representation of an English label or sign, the apostrophe -S is used as in the sentence above.

A fingerspelled name and the apostrophe -S can also be used to show the possessive but there is another way to show the possessive which does not use the apostrophe -S. An example is:

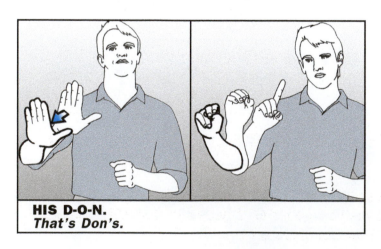

HIS D-O-N.
That's Don's.

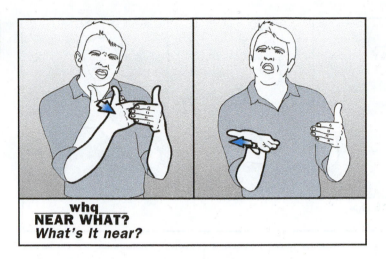

whq
NEAR WHAT?
What's it near?

16

Grammar Note

The question above asks for information about what is in the vicinity of the place being discussed. LOCALE is used to indicate an area or an approximate location as in the following:

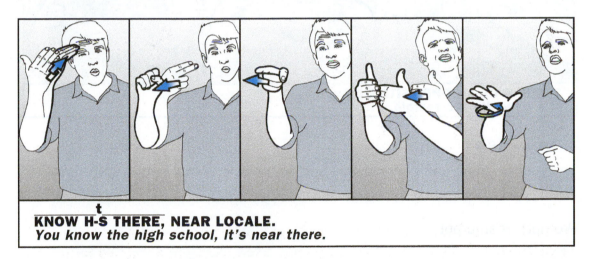

t
KNOW H-S THERE, NEAR LOCALE.
You know the high school, it's near there.

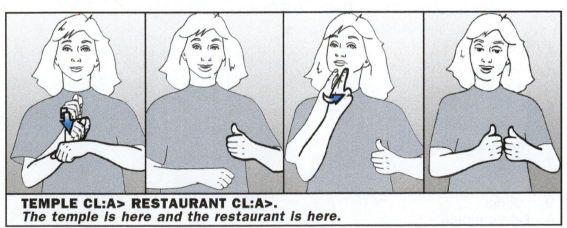

TEMPLE CL:A> RESTAURANT CL:A>.
The temple is here and the restaurant is here.

Grammar Note

In the sentence above, classifier handshapes are used to establish the location of a place and its relationship to another place (see Unit 10). Some other examples of locational relationships are:

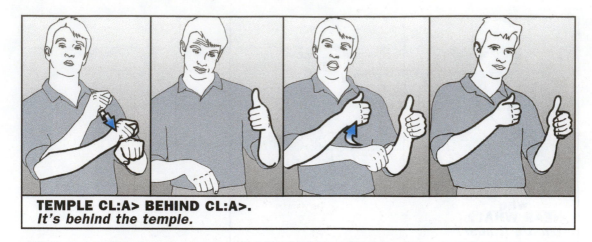

TEMPLE CL:A> BEHIND CL:A>.
It's behind the temple.

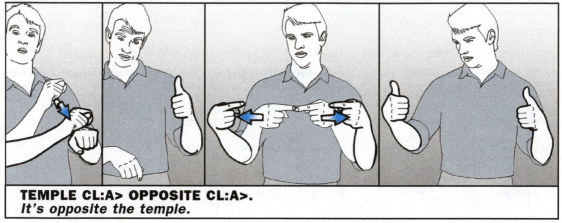

TEMPLE CL:A> OPPOSITE CL:A>.
It's opposite the temple.

Exercise 16B

Tell your partner you live opposite, next to, or behind the following. Follow the prompt.

Prompt: restaurant

RESTAURANT CL:A> OPPOSITE CL:A>.

1. post office
2. church
3. food store
4. high school
5. college
6. Marie's restaurant
7. temple
8. post office
9. college
10. Don's house

INSTRUCTIONS

Alex: MUST YOU CAREFUL. IT COMPUTER EXPENSIVE, EASY BREAK.

Lisa: O-K. I NOT KID I.

Alex: O-K. OPEN-BOX. CL:CC**-TAKE-OUT-PUT-ON TABLE. LOOK-FOR FIND

BOOK. BOOK, FOLLOW! LOOK-FOR FIND PLUG-IN-THERE. LOOK-FOR

             when

CL:L̈L̈-DISK, CL:L̈*-PUT-IN. FINISH, TURN-ON-(push button).

   ___when___

WAIT, SCREEN-ON, READY.

16

Key Structures

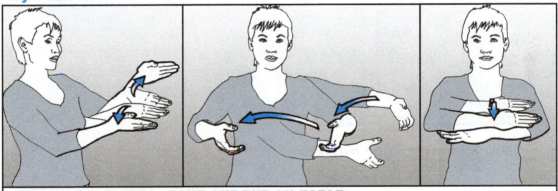

OPEN-BOX. CL:CC-TAKE-OUT-PUT-ON TABLE.**
Open the box. Take it out and put it on the table.

Grammar Note

CL:CC** in the previous sentence is the same as the instrument classifier
CL:C* in Unit 7, but the object being handled is large enough to require two
hands.

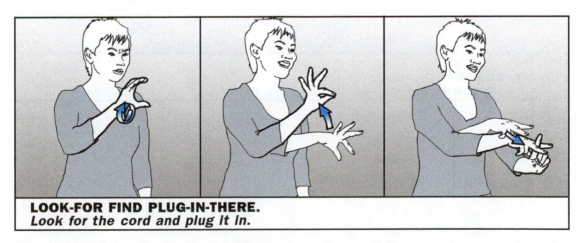

LOOK-FOR FIND PLUG-IN-THERE.
Look for the cord and plug it in.

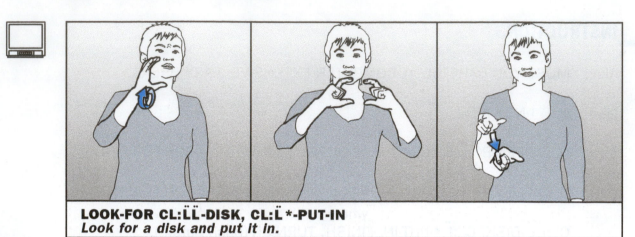

LOOK-FOR CL:ḶḶ-DISK, CL:Ḷ*-PUT-IN
Look for a disk and put it in.

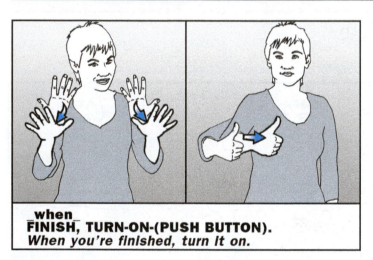

when
FINISH, TURN-ON-(PUSH BUTTON).
When you're finished, turn it on.

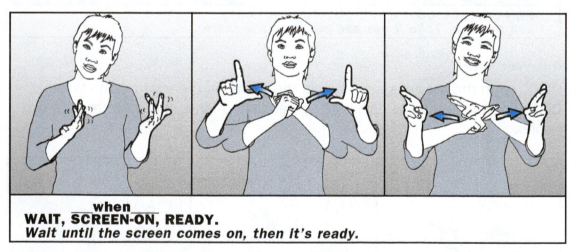

_____when_____
WAIT, SCREEN-ON, READY.
Wait until the screen comes on, then it's ready.

Exercise 16C

Take turns instructing each other how to do something, such as make a pie, paint a house, change a flat tire, or any other simple task.

VOCABULARY

▶ **For Giving Directions**

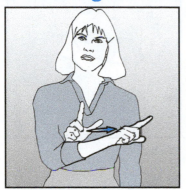

LEFT (DIR)

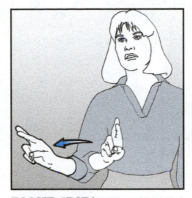

RIGHT (DIR)

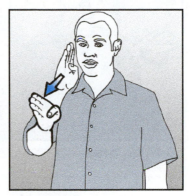

STRAIGHT

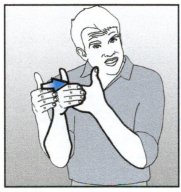

NEAR, close

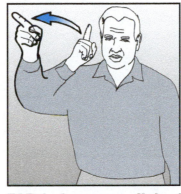

FAR-1, far away, distant

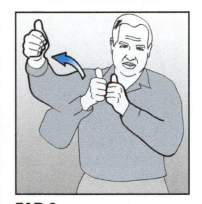

FAR-2

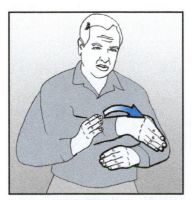

CROSS-OVER

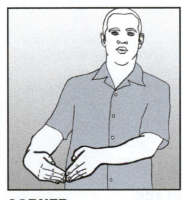

CORNER

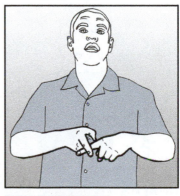

INTERSECTION, crossroads

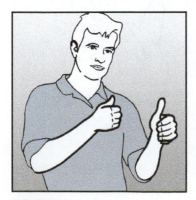

BEHIND

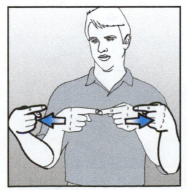

OPPOSITE

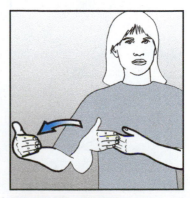

NEXT-TO, beside

16

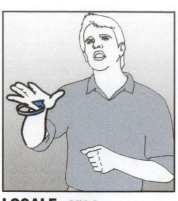

LOCALE, area

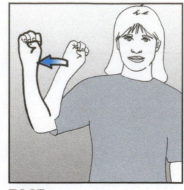

EAST

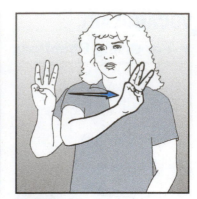

WEST

▶ **Verb Pair**

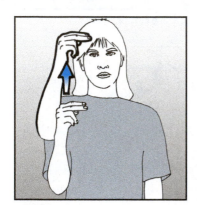

NORTH

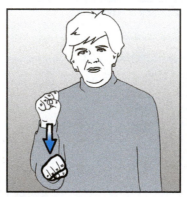

SOUTH

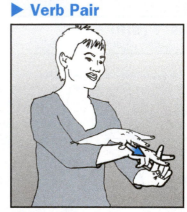

PLUG-IN

▶ **Places**

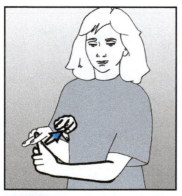

UNPLUG

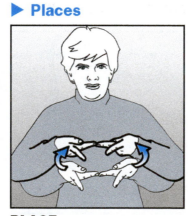

PLACE

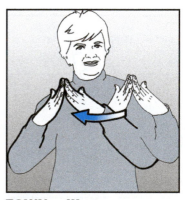

TOWN, village

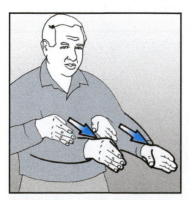

STREET, road, avenue

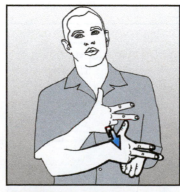

PARKING, parking lot

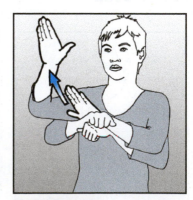

MOUNTAINS

▶ **Other Vocabulary**

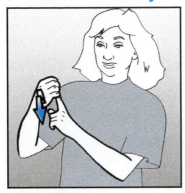

ELEVATOR

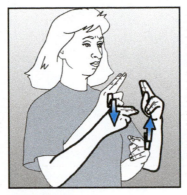

BUILDING

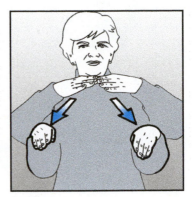

ROOF

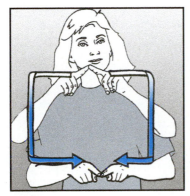

SIGN

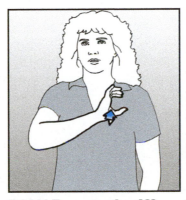

POLICE, cop, sheriff

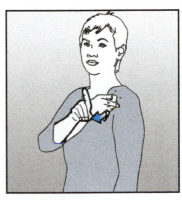

DETECTIVE

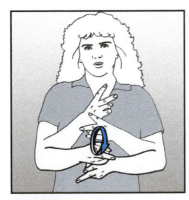

CAREFUL

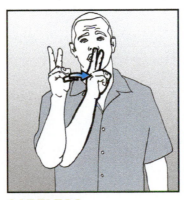

CARELESS

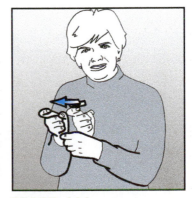

TEASE, kid

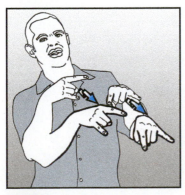

MOCK

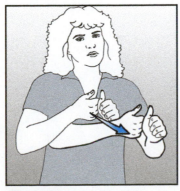

FOLLOW

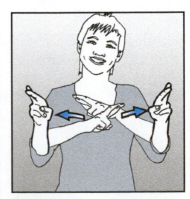

READY

16

UNIT 17

Suggestions and Advice

In this unit, you will learn to make suggestions and give advice.

You will learn the forms for EVERY-MONTH and EVERY-YEAR.

You will learn to give feedback to another signer while he/she is signing and how to use confirming signs to show you understand.

In a culture note, you will learn about the popularity of bowling in some Deaf communities.

SUGGESTIONS

                  _____whq_____
Chris: BORED I. #DO TONIGHT?

Lisa: I SUGGEST TWO, YOU CHOOSE. FIRST WHY^NOT TWO-OF-US GO-AWAY
       BOWLING. TONIGHT DEAF CL:55≋-GO-THERE.
              whq
Chris: O-K. OTHER?
       _____if_____
Lisa: BOWLING DON'T-WANT, WHY^NOT TWO-OF-US GO-AWAY MOVIE.

Chris: BOWLING EVERY-WEEK, BORED, GO-AWAY MOVIE.

Key Structures

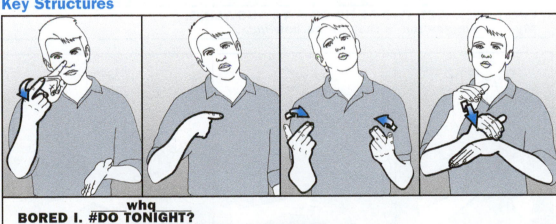

          _____whq_____
BORED I. #DO TONIGHT?
I'm bored. What do you want to do tonight?

Note

BORED is used in the previous sentence to indicate there is nothing to do of interest or, as in the last sentence of the dialogue, to express that one is tired of something.

However, BORED is also used to express, in strong terms, that one does not want to do something as in the following example:

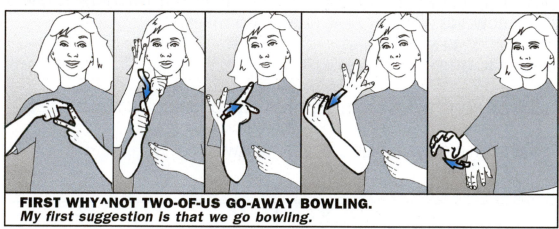

<u>   ^t   </u>
EXPLAIN AGAIN, BORED I.
I don't feel like explaining again.

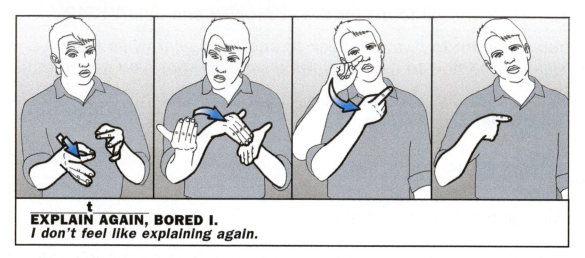

FIRST WHY^NOT TWO-OF-US GO-AWAY BOWLING.
My first suggestion is that we go bowling.

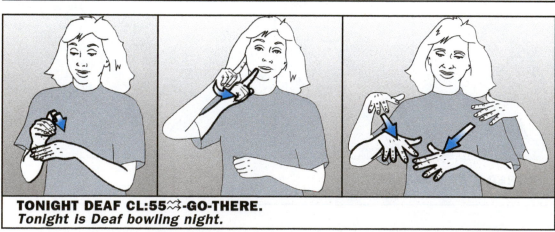

TONIGHT DEAF CL:55﹏-GO-THERE.
Tonight is Deaf bowling night.

Culture Note

The bowling night referred to in the above sentence is the weekly meeting of a local Deaf bowling league. Such leagues have been popular in many Deaf communities. There are several reasons for this popularity: the opportunity to socialize while waiting between turns, the opportunity for all to participate regardless of athletic ability, and the prize money sometimes offered to winning teams.

Also popular are the regional and national sports organizations for Deaf people. The American Amateur Association of the Deaf (AAAD) sponsors competition across the country in various sports, notably basketball and softball. The AAAD is also the governing body for the United States' entry in the World Games for the Deaf held every four years at different sites around the world.

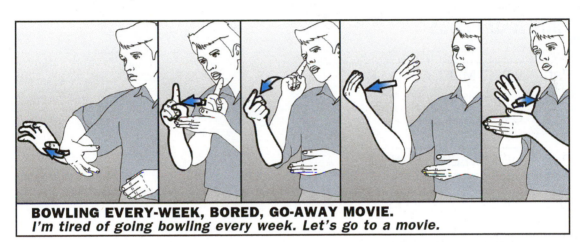

BOWLING EVERY-WEEK, BORED, GO-AWAY MOVIE.
I'm tired of going bowling every week. Let's go to a movie.

Grammar Note

The forms for EVERY-MONTH and EVERY-YEAR are as follows:

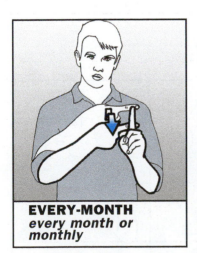

EVERY-MONTH
every month or monthly

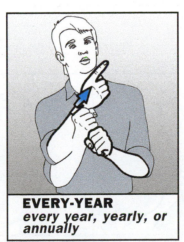

EVERY-YEAR
every year, yearly, or annually

17

Exercise 17A

Suggest to your partner and another person that the three of you do the following. Follow the prompt:

Prompt: go swimming

    WHY^NOT TWO-OF-US GO-THERE SWIM.

1. go to a restaurant
2. go skiing
3. practice signing
4. go for ice cream
5. get a captioned video

6. go for coffee
7. play tennis
8. work on computer
9. meet tomorrow
10. take up bowling

TIME AND PLACE

```
              _____q_____
Pat:   WANT MEET AGAIN, HUH?

           _whq_
Lisa:  O-K. WHEN?

           _____q_____
Pat:   NEXT-WEEK FRIDAY?

           _whq_
Lisa:  FINE. TIME?

           _____q_____
Pat:   MORNING TIME-9?

                              _____q_____
Lisa:  BETTER 11 APPROXIMATELY. YOUR HOUSE RIGHT?

Pat:   RIGHT.
```

Key Structures

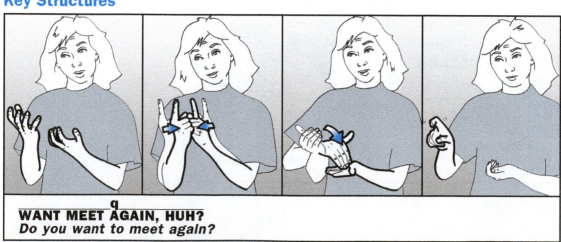

              q
WANT MEET AGAIN, HUH?
Do you want to meet again?

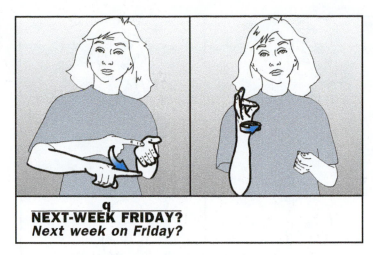

q
NEXT-WEEK FRIDAY?
Next week on Friday?

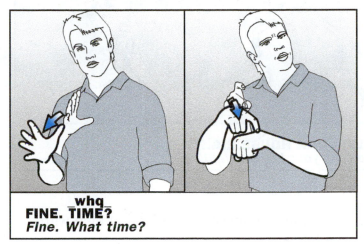

whq
FINE. TIME?
Fine. What time?

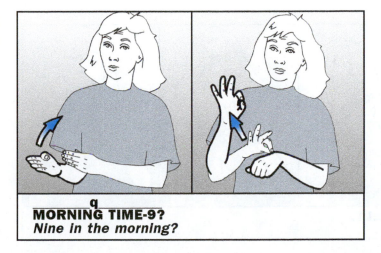

q
MORNING TIME-9?
Nine in the morning?

17

Note

In the dialogue above, note that the two signers give each other constant feedback by head nods or headshakes and frequently use confirming signs such as FINE, SURE, and O-K as they question each other about specific information.

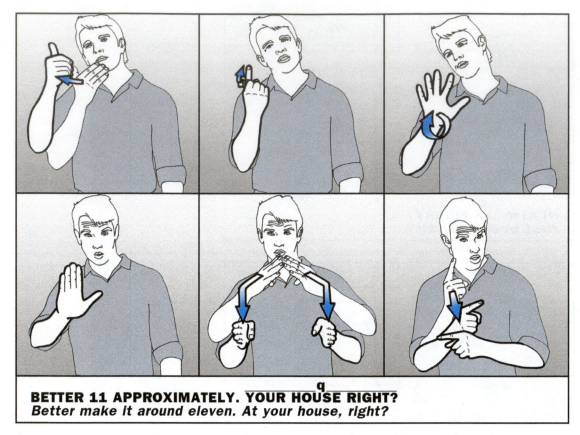

BETTER 11 APPROXIMATELY. $\overline{\text{YOUR HOUSE}}^{\text{q}}\overline{\text{RIGHT?}}$
Better make it around eleven. At your house, right?

Note

APPROXIMATELY is used with time as in the above sentence and also with age and money amounts as in the following:

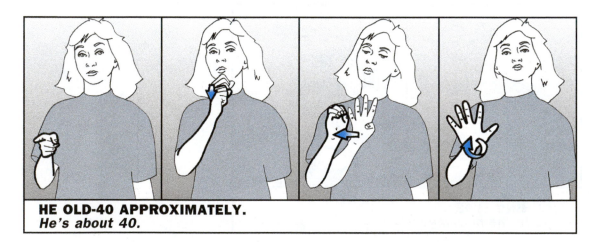

HE OLD-40 APPROXIMATELY.
He's about 40.

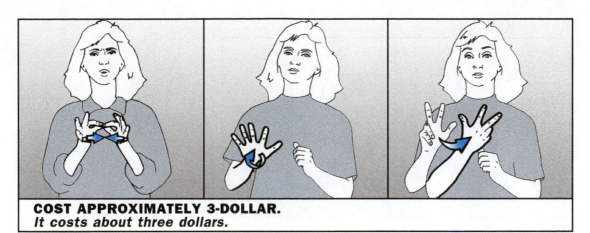

COST APPROXIMATELY 3-DOLLAR.
It costs about three dollars.

Exercise 17B

Suggest the following times and places to meet your partner. Each of you should ask for and give confirmation to make sure you agree.

1. Saturday, 3:30, here
2. next month, same time, your partner's house
3. next week, Tuesday, 8:00, your house
4. Mondays, 1:00, at the club
5. every week, Wednesdays, 5:30, in the library
6. Thursday morning, 7:30, on the corner near your house
7. in two weeks, 12:00, at the high school
8. next Friday, 8:00, in L.A.
9. everyday, noon, in my room
10. every morning, 6:00, at the coffee place on the corner

ADVICE

```
                              _whq_
Pat:    MONEY NOT-YET ARRIVE. #DO I?
```

```
             _____q_____
Chris:  FINISH YOU-PAGE-HER?
```

Pat: I-PAGE-HER BEFORE MONDAY. SHE-TOLD-ME I WILL GET TODAY.

```
                _____q_____
        SHOULD I-T-T-Y-HER AGAIN, HUH?
```

Chris: BETTER NOT. MAYBE GO-AHEAD GET LAWYER.

```
                _____q_____
Pat:    SHOULD I I-TELL-HER I GET LAWYER O-R...?
```

Chris: BETTER SAY NOTHING. YOU-ASK-HER LAWYER.

Key Structures

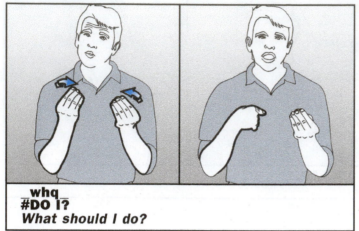

whq
#DO I?
What should I do?

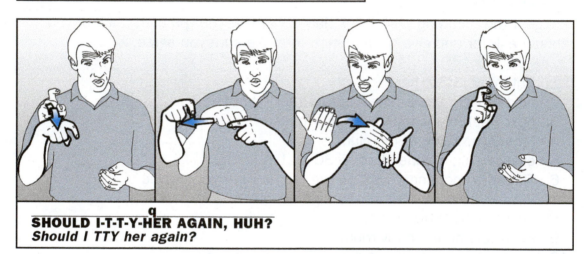

q
SHOULD I-T-T-Y-HER AGAIN, HUH?
Should I TTY her again?

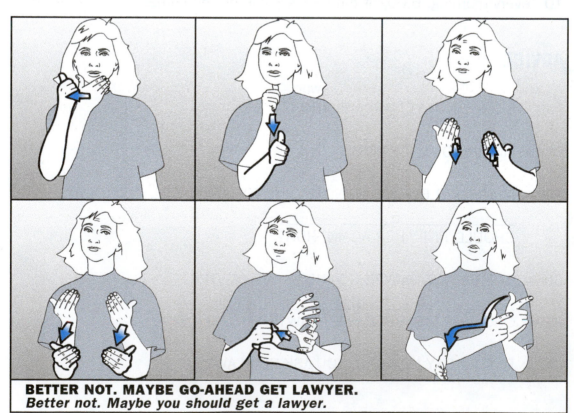

BETTER NOT. MAYBE GO-AHEAD GET LAWYER.
Better not. Maybe you should get a lawyer.

Grammar Note

Sentences that contain advice are often preceded by SHOULD, BETTER (NOT), ADVISE, WARN, SUGGEST, or MAYBE as in the sentence above.

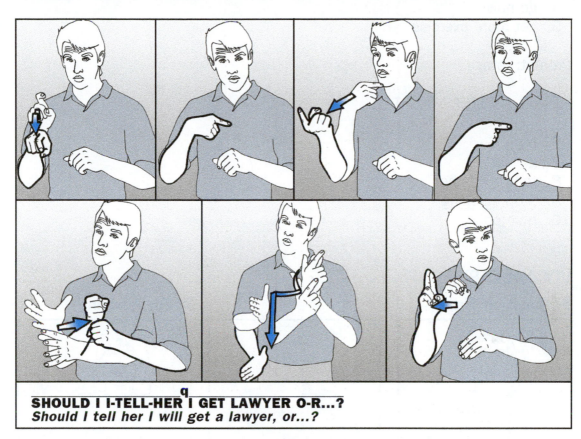

> q
> **SHOULD I I-TELL-HER I GET LAWYER O-R...?**
> *Should I tell her I will get a lawyer, or...?*

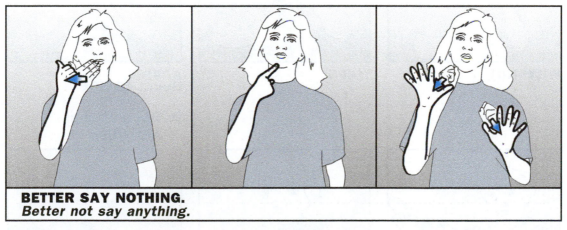

BETTER SAY NOTHING.
Better not say anything.

Exercise 17C

Give the following advice. Follow the prompt.

Prompt: rest more

        SHOULD YOU MORE REST.

17

1. eat less
2. tell your mother
3. take it easy
4. go now
5. get more exercise

Prompt: stay

> BETTER YOU STAY.

6. hurry
7. get up
8. tell your father
9. stop smoking
10. quit job

VOCABULARY

▶ **Question Signs**

▶ **For Advising**

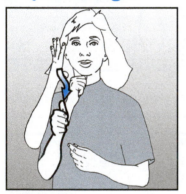

WHY^NOT

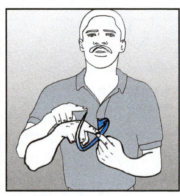

WHEN

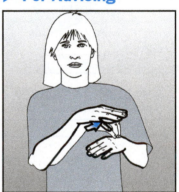

**ADVISE,
Noun: ADVICE**

▶ **Recreational
Activities**

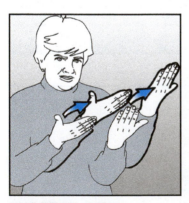

**SUGGEST, offer,
propose**

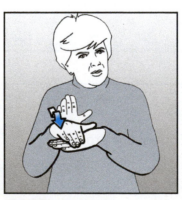

WARN, caution

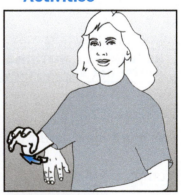

BOWLING

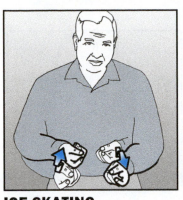

ICE-SKATING

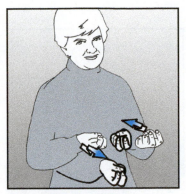

ROLLER-SKATING

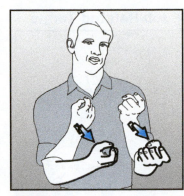

SKIING

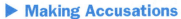

▶ **Making Accusations**

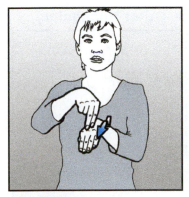

SURFING

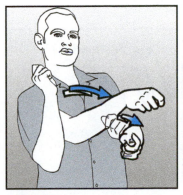

FISHING

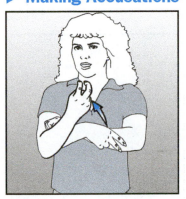

STEAL

17

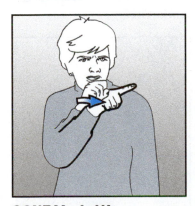

SQUEAL, tattle

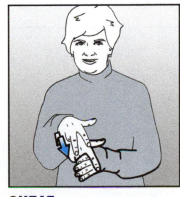

CHEAT

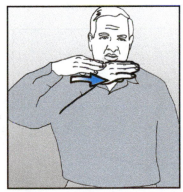

LIE

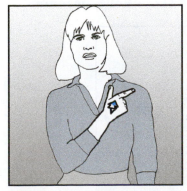

LAZY

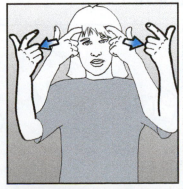

ARROGANT, egotistical, conceited

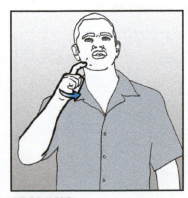

JEALOUS

▶ **Job-Related Terms**

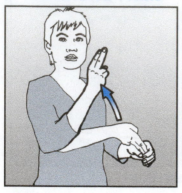

QUIT

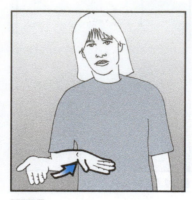

HIRE

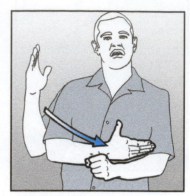

TERMINATE, fire

▶ **Other Vocabulary**

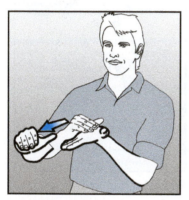

LAY-OFF, release

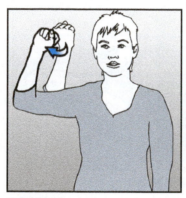

STRIKE

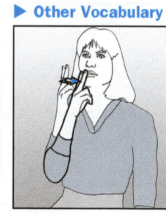

SMOKING

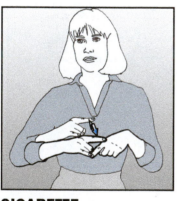

CIGARETTE

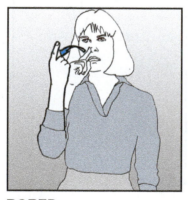

BORED

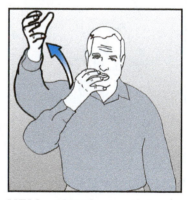

YELL, shout, scream

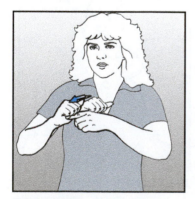

PRACTICE, exercise

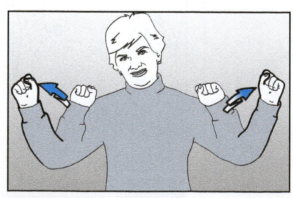

EXERCISE (physical)

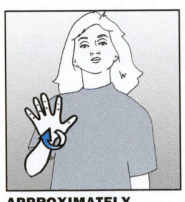

APPROXIMATELY

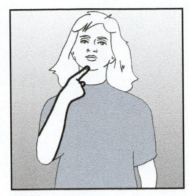

SAY

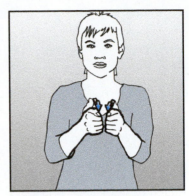

PAGE, use pager

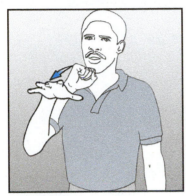

NOTHING

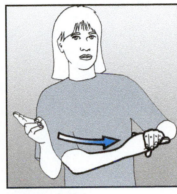

GO-TO-BED

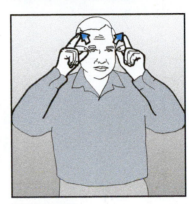

WAKE-UP

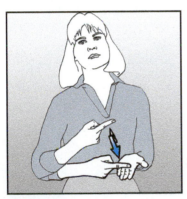

DISCUSS

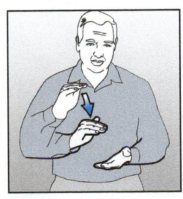

LESS

17

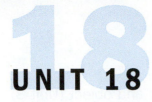

UNIT 18

Attitudes and Opinions

In this unit, you will learn how to express attitudes, values, and opinions as well as learn to ask what others think.

You will learn about verbs that change their movement to show more than one subject or object.

You will also learn to use quantifiers such as MANY and SOME with different kinds of nouns.

WHAT OTHERS THINK

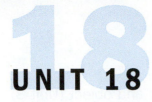

Lisa: _____t_____ _____q_____
I I-ASK-YOU-TWO. FOOD HERE, YOU THINK GOOD?

Alex: _____whq_____
WHAT-FOR YOU-ASK-ME?

Lisa: ___q___
TWO-OF-YOU FREQUENT HERE. RIGHT?

Alex: _____whq_____
RIGHT. WHY YOU WANT KNOW?

Lisa: COLLEGE NEWSPAPER I WRITE ARTICLE, PRINT.

Alex: _____q_____
USE OUR NAME?

Lisa: _q_ ____t____ ____q____
NONE NAME. O-K? FOOD HERE, LIKE YOU?

Key Structures

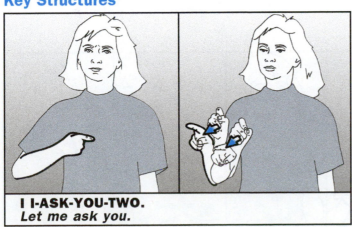

I I-ASK-YOU-TWO.
Let me ask you.

Grammar Note

Some verbs which change their movement to show subject and object (Unit 3) can show:

a. TWO, dual subjects or objects as in the previous sentence (I-ASK-YOU-TWO).

b. EACH, several subjects or objects as in the following examples:

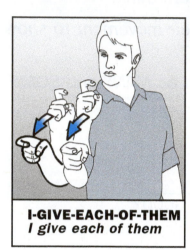
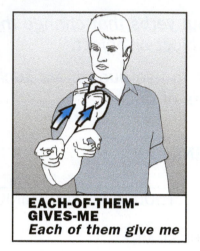

I-GIVE-EACH-OF-THEM
I give each of them

EACH-OF-THEM-GIVES-ME
Each of them give me

c. However, ALL can be used only with objects as in the following examples:

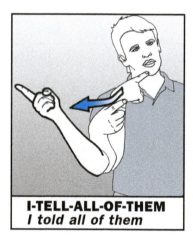

I-TELL-ALL-OF-THEM
I told all of them

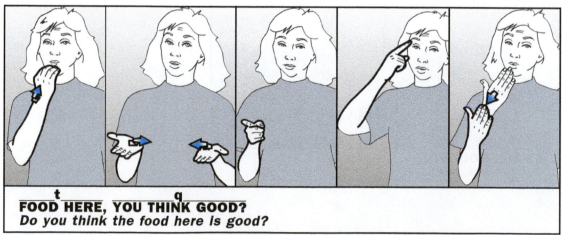

<u>   t   q   </u>
FOOD HERE, YOU THINK GOOD?
Do you think the food here is good?

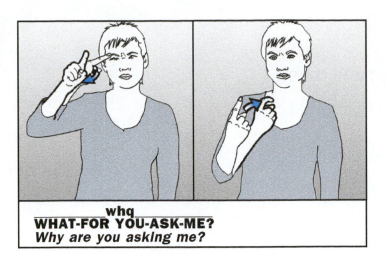

whq
WHAT-FOR YOU-ASK-ME?
Why are you asking me?

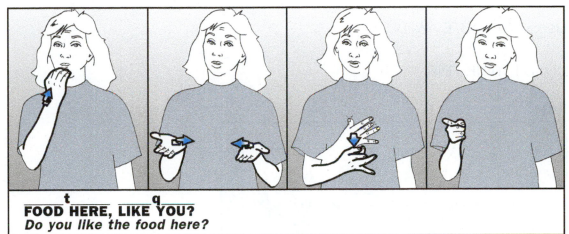

t _____ q _____
FOOD HERE, LIKE YOU?
Do you like the food here?

18

Exercise 18A

Ask your partner her/his opinion of the following. Follow the prompt.

Prompt: the new president

_____t_____ ____whq____   ____q____
KNOW YOU NEW PRESIDENT, THINK YOU? or LIKE YOU?

1. a book (name a book you read)
2. a movie (name a movie you saw recently)
3. the city you live in
4. the shirt or dress you are wearing
5. a make of car (name a car, i.e., Honda)
6. a movie or pop star (name someone)
7. his/her mother's cooking
8. the local newspaper (give name)
9. a magazine (name a magazine)
10. your hairstyle

OPINIONS

Lisa: ODD. MAKE P-I-Z-Z-A, TASTE LOUSY.

          whq __whq__
Chris: WHY? WRONG?

Lisa: DON'T-KNOW I. TASTE IT.

(Chris tastes it.)

Chris: DELICIOUS!

Lisa: NO! TASTE AWFUL.

Chris: I THINK FINE.

Key Structures

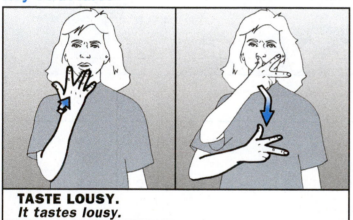

TASTE LOUSY.
It tastes lousy.

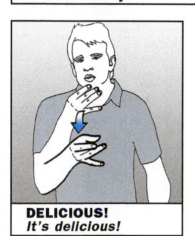

DELICIOUS!
It's delicious!

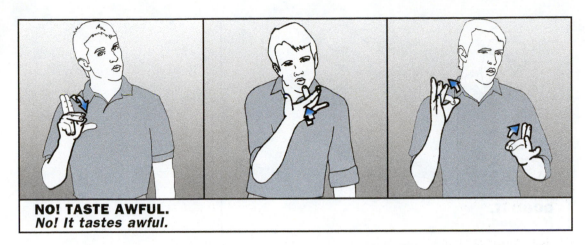

NO! TASTE AWFUL.
No! It tastes awful.

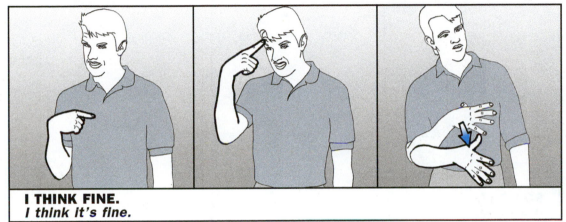

I THINK FINE.
I think it's fine.

18

Note

The previous sentences are some of the possible ways to express an opinion about food or other things. Some other ways to express an opinion are:

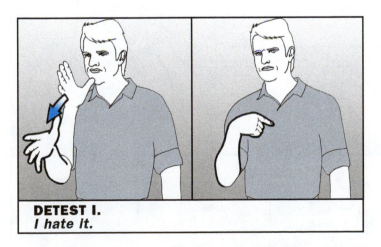

DETEST I.
I hate it.

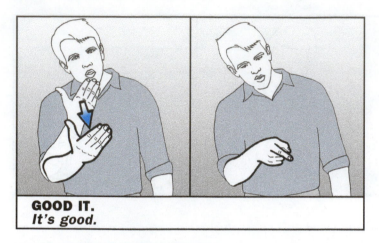

GOOD IT.
It's good.

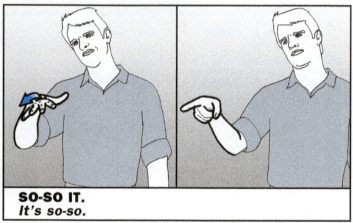

SO-SO IT.
It's so-so.

Examples of opinions about something other than food are:

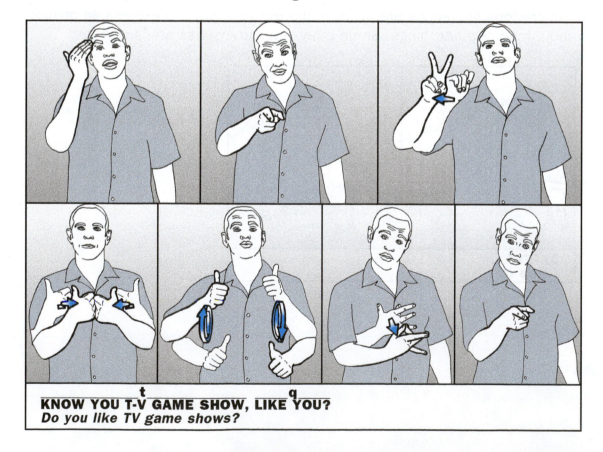

KNOW YOU T-V GAME SHOW, LIKE YOU?
Do you like TV game shows?

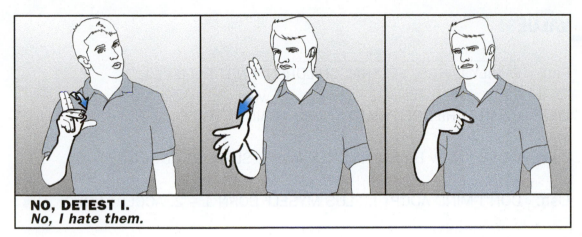

NO, DETEST I.
No, I hate them.

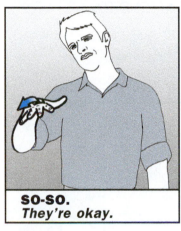

SO-SO.
They're okay.

18

Exercise 18B

Name a specific item or title from the following categories and express an opinion about it. Give positive, negative, or average opinions. Follow the prompt.

Prompt: a movie

<u>   t   </u>
MOVIE D-R-A-C-U-L-A, GOOD.

1. a movie
2. a food
3. a city
4. a television show
5. a vegetable
6. a make of car
7. a movie or pop star
8. a course
9. a type of work
10. a restaurant

VALUES

_____t_____
Pat: FAMILY LARGE, SEVERAL CHILDREN, I NOT BELIEVE I.

_____whq_____
Lisa: I WANT CHILDREN MANY I. WHY AGAINST YOU?

Pat: WORLD NOW HAVE CHILDREN MANY. SUPPORT ADOPT I.

_____q_____
Lisa: DON'T-MIND ADOPT I, PLUS MYSELF BORN 1 – 2. ACCEPT YOU?

Pat: ACCEPT I. I BELIEVE STRONG MUST CHILDREN ATTEND-TO.

Lisa: RIGHT. AGREE 100 PERCENT.

Key Structures

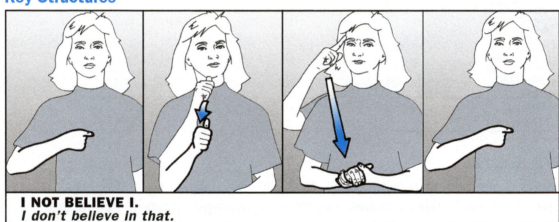

I NOT BELIEVE I.
I don't believe in that.

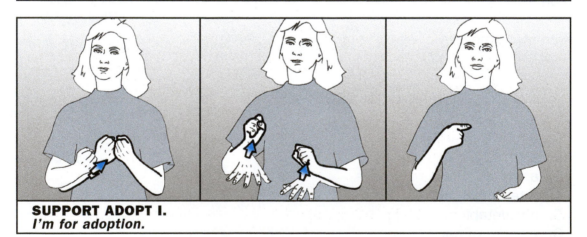

SUPPORT ADOPT I.
I'm for adoption.

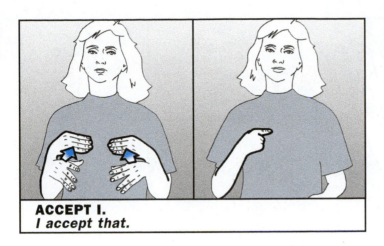

ACCEPT I.
I accept that.

Note

Opposing values are expressed in the sentences above and other sentences in the preceding dialogue. They are summarized here:

BELIEVE STRONG I.	NOT BELIEVE I.
SUPPORT I.	AGAINST I.
ACCEPT I.	NOT ACCEPT I.

18

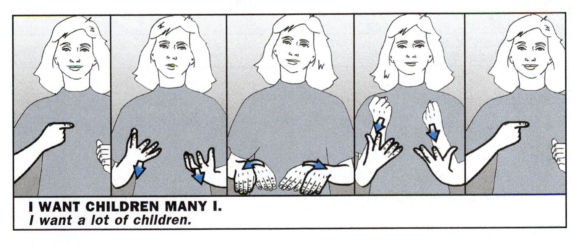

I WANT CHILDREN MANY I.
I want a lot of children.

Grammar Note

Quantifiers such as MANY, SEVERAL, A-FEW, and SOME, appear either before or after a noun (Unit 7). These quantifiers are used with count nouns such as BOOK, CAR, STUDENT, and CHILDREN.

Additional quantifiers which appear with non-count nouns such as FOOD, MILK, MONEY are: PLENTY, SOME, and A-LITTLE, as in the following:

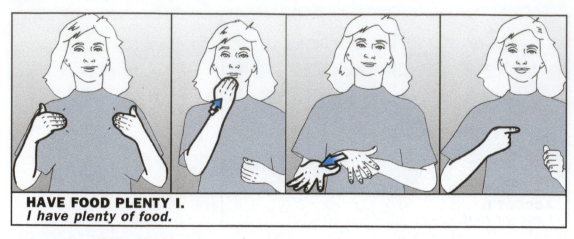

HAVE FOOD PLENTY I.
I have plenty of food.

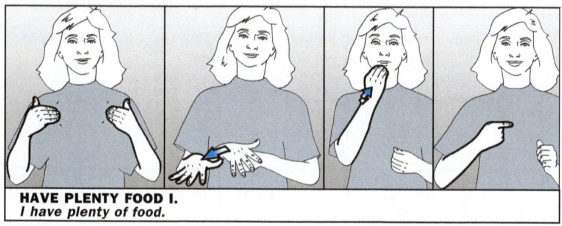

HAVE PLENTY FOOD I.
I have plenty of food.

Exercise 18C

Use one of the quantifiers above with the following. Follow the prompt.

Prompt: chairs

       HAVE CHAIR MANY.

1. furniture
2. pictures
3. water
4. experience
5. money
6. children
7. houses
8. stores
9. shoes
10. paper

VOCABULARY

▶ Opinion and Attitude Signs

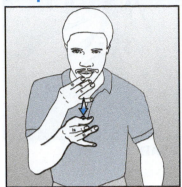

DELICIOUS

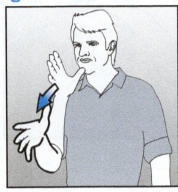

DETEST

▶ Expressing Values

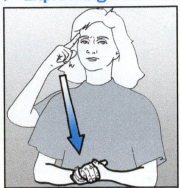

BELIEVE

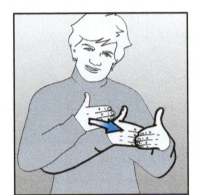

AGAINST, opposed, con

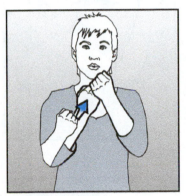

SUPPORT, pro

▶ Quantifiers

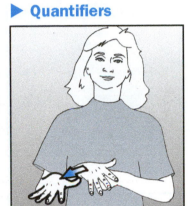

PLENTY

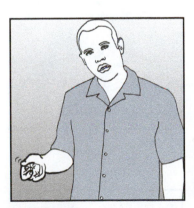

A-LITTLE

▶ Astronomy

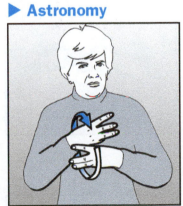

WORLD

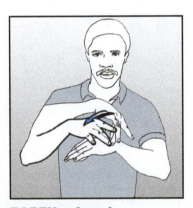

EARTH, planet

18

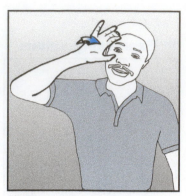

SUN

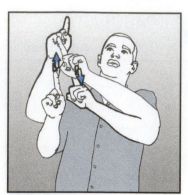

MOON

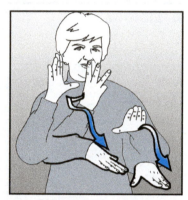

STAR

▶ The Earth

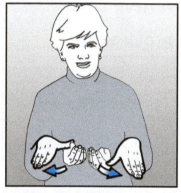

LAND

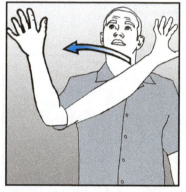

SKY

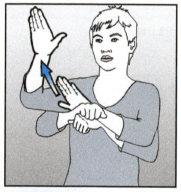

OCEAN, sea

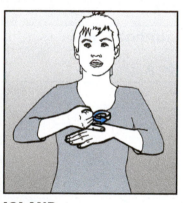

MOUNTAIN

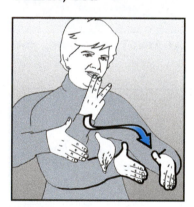

ISLAND

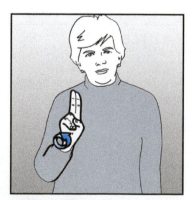

RIVER

▶ Other Vocabulary

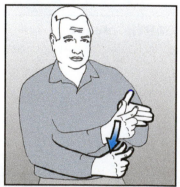

ARTICLE, column

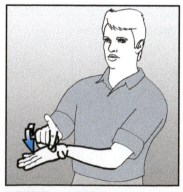

PRINT, publish

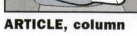

USE, wear

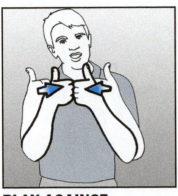

**PLAY-AGAINST,
Noun: GAME**

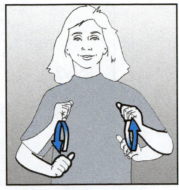

**SHOW, play, drama,
act, theater**

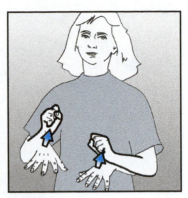

ADOPT

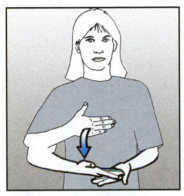

**BORN, give birth to,
birth**

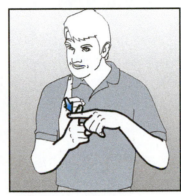

PLUS, in addition

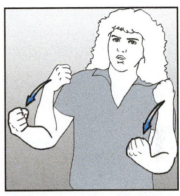

STRONG, predominant

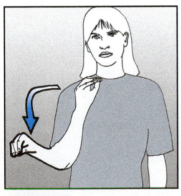

PERCENT

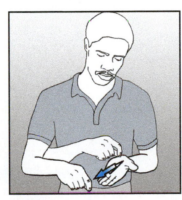

WRITE

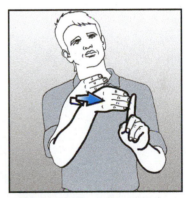

FREQUENT, patronize

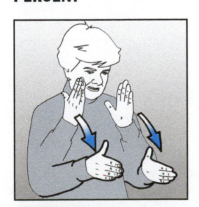

**ATTEND-TO, pay
attention to, focus on**

18

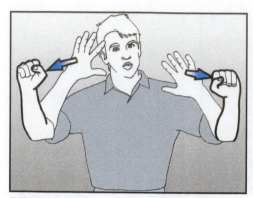

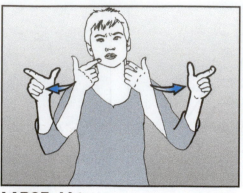

PRESIDENT, superintendent, chancellor

LARGE, big

UNIT 19

Recreational Activities

In this unit, you will learn to talk about activities and describe a sequence of activities.

You will learn how to inflect some verbs to show REPEATEDLY and CONTINUALLY and the facial adverbials that accompany these inflections.

You will also learn reduplication to form the plural of some nouns to indicate "all over the place" or "everywhere."

ACTIVITIES

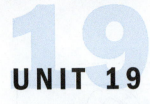

```
              ____q_____
Alex:   SKI LIKE YOU?

                   ___t___
Pat:    CRAZY-ABOUT. WINTER, I GO-THERE-REPEATEDLY.

        _____whq_____
Alex:   WHERE FREQUENT YOU?

Pat:    B-I-G B-E-A-R. NEAR. I DRIVE-THERE EASY.

        _____q_____
Alex:   SNOW CL:BB-THICK-LAYER?

Pat:    YES, CL:BB-THICK-LAYER. NICE. NOT CL:55≋ PEOPLE.

        _____if_____  ____q____
Alex:   YOU GO-THERE, I JOIN-YOU?

Pat:    SURE.
```

Key Structures

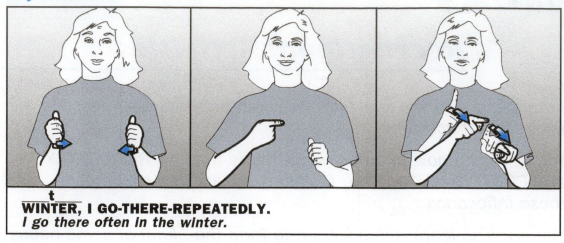

$\overline{\text{WINTER,}}^{\text{t}}$ I GO-THERE-REPEATEDLY.
I go there often in the winter.

Grammar Note

Some verbs showing action can repeat their movement to show that the action is done frequently, repeatedly, or regularly as in GO-THERE-REPEATEDLY above.

The following facial adverbs are often used with these verbs to show the manner in which an action is done.

a.   Mouth opening and closing, to show intensity or effort:

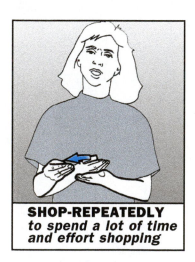

SHOP-REPEATEDLY
to spend a lot of time and effort shopping

b. Lips pursed to show lack of intensity or effort, ease:

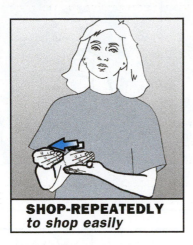

SHOP-REPEATEDLY
to shop easily

c. Lips pursed together and eyebrows squeezed together to show diligence, care, or deliberation:

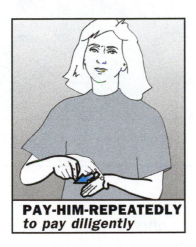

PAY-HIM-REPEATEDLY
to pay diligently

19

d. Tongue slightly protruding through pursed lips to show carelessness or lack of deliberation:

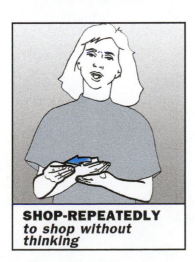

SHOP-REPEATEDLY
to shop without thinking

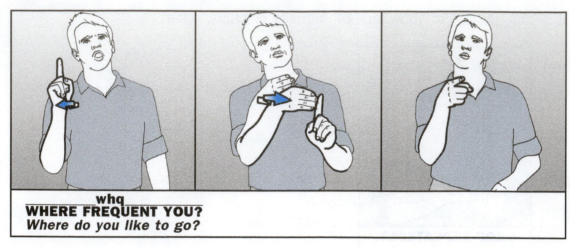

whq
WHERE FREQUENT YOU?
Where do you like to go?

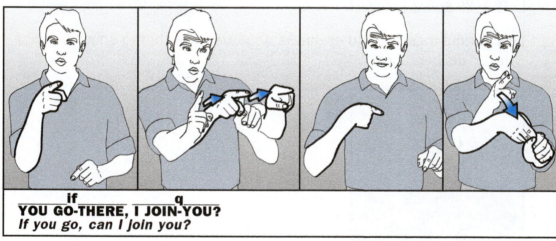

if   q
YOU GO-THERE, I JOIN-YOU?
If you go, can I join you?

Exercise 19A

Tell your partner that you do the following activities often or regularly. Use the facial adverb specified. Follow the prompt.

Prompt: skiing (diligently)

EVERY-WEEK SKI-REPEATEDLY I.

1. buy (carelessly)
2. pay (with effort)
3. tell (with effort)
4. go there (easily)
5. give (carelessly)
6. send (carefully)
7. call by TTY (with effort)

A SEQUENCE OF ACTIVITIES

Alex: _____whq_____
RECENT WEEKEND #DO YOU?

Chris: GROUP GO-AWAY B-E-A-C-H. ARRIVE EARLY TAKE-OVER PLACE. SET-UP

VOLLEYBALL. PLAY-CONTINUALLY TWO-HOUR, FINISH, DIVE-IN WATER

SWIM. FINISH, HUNGRY, COOK HOT-DOG, HAMBURGER, EAT-

CONTINUALLY. FINISH, LIE-DOWN SUN, SLEEP. LATER WAKE-UP, SWIM,

FINISH, PLAY THROW-FRISBEE. DARK, LIGHT-UP FIRE, CL:V̈V̈-SIT-IN-

CIRCLE CHAT.

Alex: WOW! FUN!

Key Structures

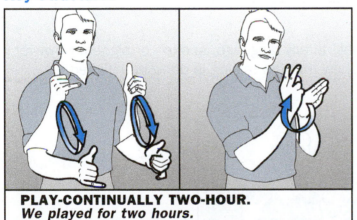

PLAY-CONTINUALLY TWO-HOUR.
We played for two hours.

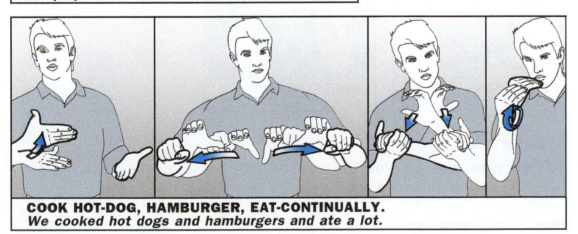

COOK HOT-DOG, HAMBURGER, EAT-CONTINUALLY.
We cooked hot dogs and hamburgers and ate a lot.

19

Grammar Note

Some verbs can change their movement to show that an action continues for a longer period of time or that something is done a lot. This is done by changing the movement to a repeating, circular movement as in PLAY-CONTINUALLY and EAT-CONTINUALLY in the previous sentences.

The facial adverbs used with REPEATEDLY are also used with CONTINUALLY.

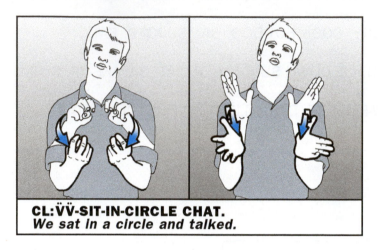

CL:V̈V̈-SIT-IN-CIRCLE CHAT.
We sat in a circle and talked.

Note

CHAT is used to mean "to chat" in any language, spoken or signed. However, two other signs are used to show that the talking is done in a signed language only:

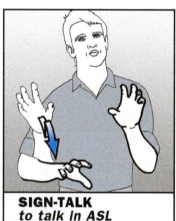

SIGN-TALK
to talk in ASL

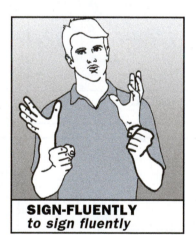

SIGN-FLUENTLY
to sign fluently

Exercise 19B

Tell your partner that you did the following activities for a long period of time. Use the facial adverb specified. Follow the prompt.

Prompt: eat hamburgers (intensively)

        _____t_____

        HAMBURGER I EAT-CONTINUALLY.

1. eat hot dogs (easily)
2. eat hot dogs (with effort)
3. play volleyball (intensively)
4. play volleyball (with pleasure)
5. work on Saturdays (intensively)
6. call by TTY (intensively)
7. run everyday (diligently)

SEASONAL ACTIVITIES

Pat: AUTUMN CAN'T WAIT, TREE++ CHANGE COLOR. WILL I GO-THERE MOUNTAIN WALK THROUGH.

Lisa: SAME-AS-YOU. WILL CAMPING I.

Pat: 1 I COMPLAIN, AUTUMN FEEL SHORT. 1-WEEK, 2-WEEK FINISH.

Lisa: TRUE BUT SNOW, LIKE I. CAN SKI C-C I.

                        _____q_____
Pat: TRUE, FUN. YOU PLAY BASKETBALL YOU?

                 _____if_____
Lisa: SOMETIMES. I JOIN TEAM, I PLAY.

Key Structures

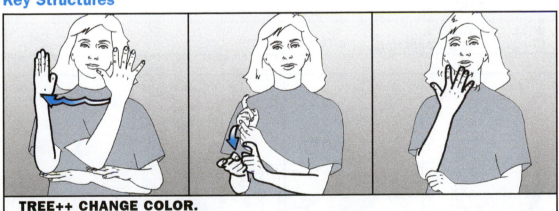

TREE++ CHANGE COLOR.
The trees will change color.

19

Grammar Note

The plural may be added to some nouns to indicate "all over the place" or "everywhere" by reduplicating the sign several times as it is moved in a sideways sweep as in TREE++ in the previous sentence. This plural form of the noun is indicated by the symbol ++. Some other examples are:

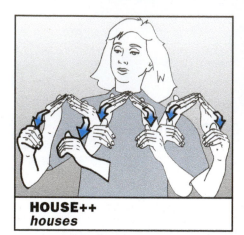

HOUSE++
houses

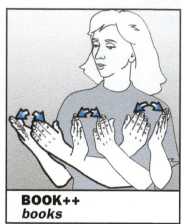

BOOK++
books

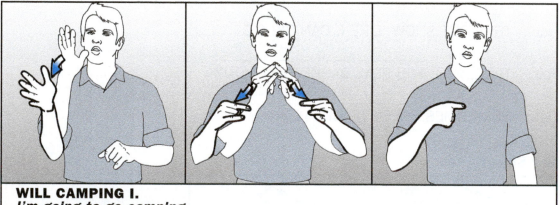

WILL CAMPING I.
I'm going to go camping.

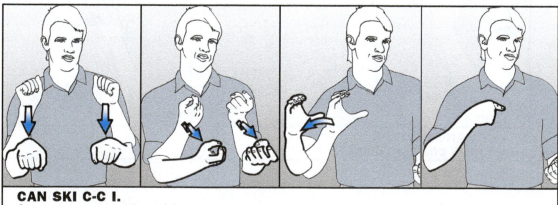

CAN SKI C-C I.
I can cross-country ski.

Exercise 19C

Tell your partner that you saw the following. Follow the prompt.

Prompt: trees

      I SEE TREE++.

1. houses
2. books
3. shoes
4. chairs
5. boxes
6. pictures
7. parked cars
8. cups
9. windows
10. tall buildings

VOCABULARY

▶ **Seasons**

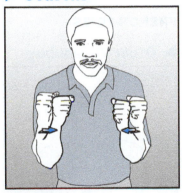

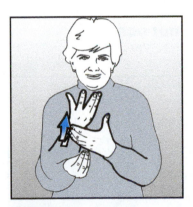

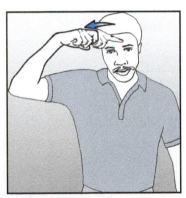

WINTER, cold   **SPRING**   **SUMMER**

▶ **Games and Activities**

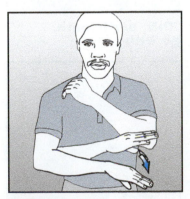

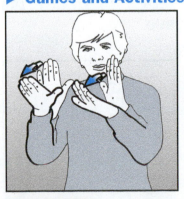

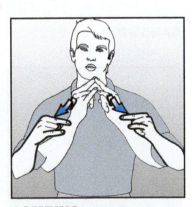

AUTUMN, fall   **VOLLEYBALL**   **CAMPING, camp**

19

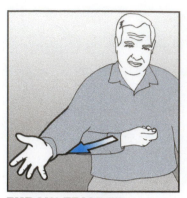

THROW-FRISBEE

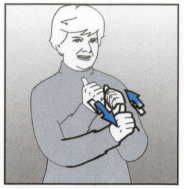

RACE, compete

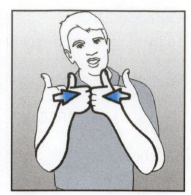

MATCH, play against

▶ **Picnic Food**

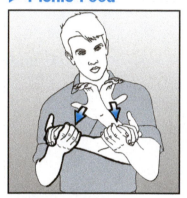

HAMBURGER

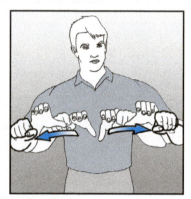

HOT-DOG

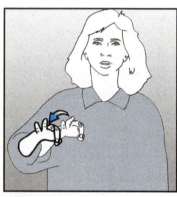

FRENCH-FRIES

▶ **Other Vocabulary**

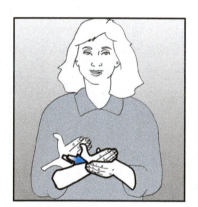

SANDWICH

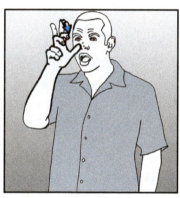

BUG

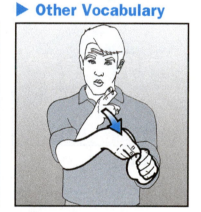

JOIN, participate, go with

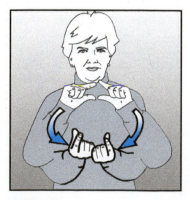

GROUP

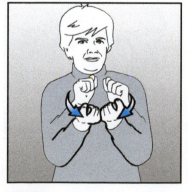

TEAM

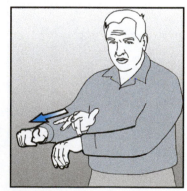

EARLY

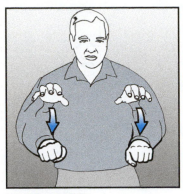

TAKE-OVER

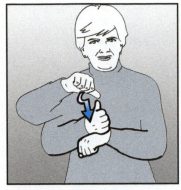

SET-UP, establish, found, erect

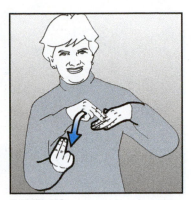

DIVE-IN

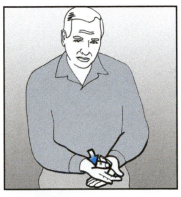

LIE-DOWN

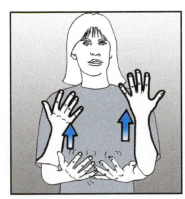

DARK

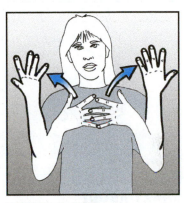

LIGHT, bright

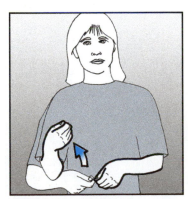

LIGHT-UP, ignite

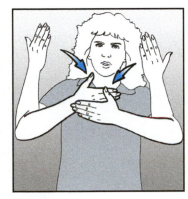

FIRE, flame

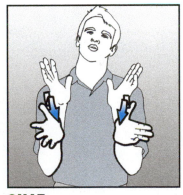

CHAT

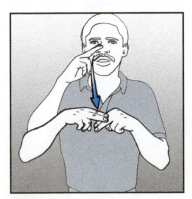

FUN

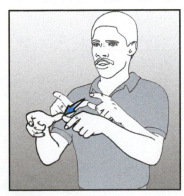

RUN

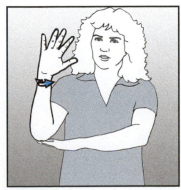

TREE

19

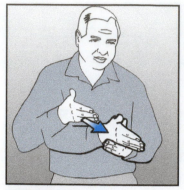

THROUGH

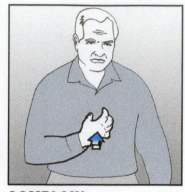

COMPLAIN

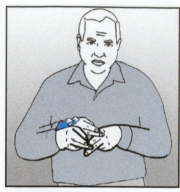

SHORT, temporary

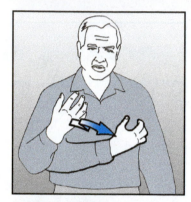

CRAZY-ABOUT

UNIT 20

Travel—Places and Experiences

In this unit, you will learn to talk about places and your travel experiences.

You will learn about adjectives that change their movement to show both REPEATEDLY and CONTINUALLY.

You will also learn about changing the movement of adjectives to show intensity.

TRAVEL EXPERIENCE

Lisa: TWO-WEEK-AGO I DRIVE-THERE WASHINGTON. PARENTS WANT JOIN-ME. I SAY-OKAY. TWO-OF-THEM EXCITED. THREE-OF-US LEAVE TUESDAY MORNING NONE PROBLEM. LATER STOP LUNCH. MOTHER ALWAYS REMIND FATHER TAKE-PILL. MOTHER WORRY-REPEATEDLY FATHER HEART. FATHER DON'T-WANT TAKE-PILL.

_____if_____
#IF MOTHER SHE-REMIND-HIM-REPEATEDLY, FATHER DETEST. I KNOW^THAT SINCE PARENTS TEND-TO QUARREL. I EMBARRASSED-REPEATEDLY. FINALLY QUIET. FROM-THEN-ON O-K.

_____q_____
Alex: RELIEVED YOU?

Lisa: (emphatic) YES!

Key Structures

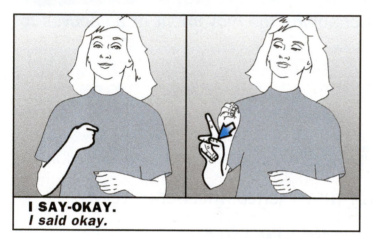

PARENTS WANT JOIN-ME.
My parents wanted to come with me.

I SAY-OKAY.
I said okay.

Grammar Note

In the two sentences above, there are two verbs that change their movement to show subject and object, JOIN and SAY-OKAY. Note that when there is a multiple subject or object such as MOTHER AND FATHER or PARENTS which are thought of as a unit, they are treated as a single subject or object.

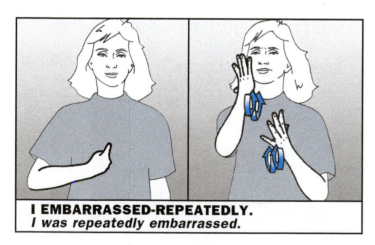

I EMBARRASSED-REPEATEDLY.
I was repeatedly embarrassed.

Grammar Note

Some adjectives repeat their movement to show that a state occurs again and again over a period of time as in the state of being embarrassed above, EMBARRASSED-REPEATEDLY. Another example of this is:

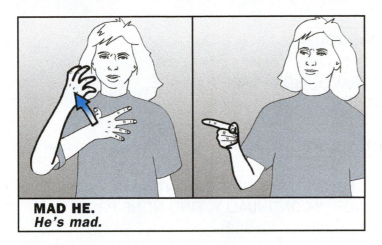

MAD HE.
He's mad.

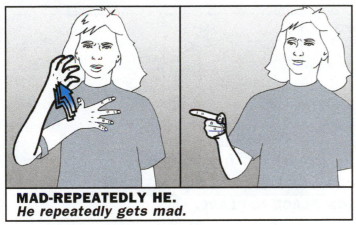

MAD-REPEATEDLY HE.
He repeatedly gets mad.

Exercise 20A

Tell your partner that the following occurs repeatedly. Follow the prompt.

Prompt: worry

      WORRY-REPEATEDLY I.

1. mad
2. embarrassed
3. sick
4. frustrated
5. wrong
6. late
7. careless
8. disappointed
9. depressed
10. stupid

20

MORE TRAVEL EXPERIENCE

Alex: NEVER FORGET I GO-THERE EUROPE. TRAVEL-AROUND-CONTINUALLY TWO-MONTH I.

                                    q
Pat: TRAVEL-AROUND ALONE YOU?

Alex: YES. I GET-ON TRAIN TRAVEL-FROM-PLACE-TO-PLACE. MEET-REPEATEDLY DEAF.

                                    q
Pat: WOW. WISH I GO-WITH I. TRAVEL-AROUND SMOOTH?

Alex: YES. FRIEND SHE-TELL-ME SHE FRUSTRATED-CONTINUALLY, CAN'T FIND PLACE SLEEP. I WORRY-CONTINUALLY, FIND NONE PROBLEM.

Key Structures

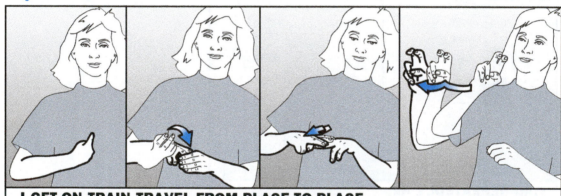

I GET-ON TRAIN TRAVEL-FROM-PLACE-TO-PLACE.
I got around on the train.

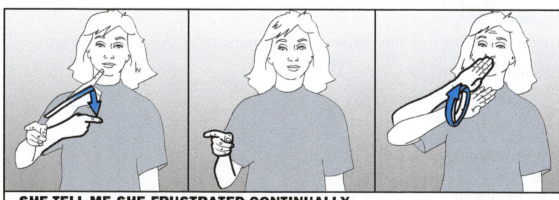

SHE-TELL-ME SHE FRUSTRATED-CONTINUALLY.
She told me she was always frustrated.

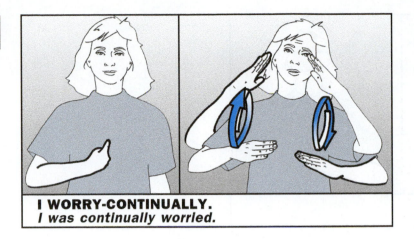

I WORRY-CONTINUALLY.
I was continually worried.

Grammar Note

In these two preceding sentences, the adjectives FRUSTRATED and WORRY have a repeated, circular movement to show that the state continues for a period of time. Some other examples of adjectives that change to show a continued state are:

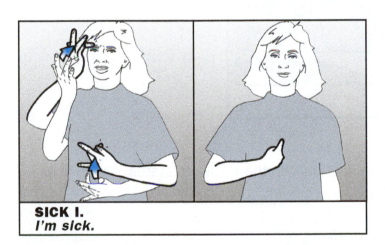

SICK I.
I'm sick.

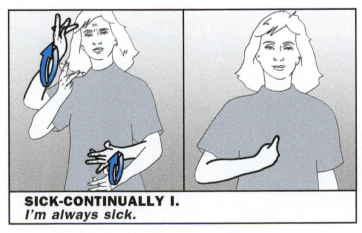

SICK-CONTINUALLY I.
I'm always sick.

20

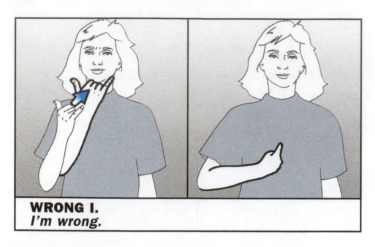

WRONG I.
I'm wrong.

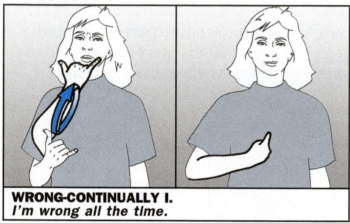

WRONG-CONTINUALLY I.
I'm wrong all the time.

Exercise 20B

Tell your partner that you are continually in the following states. Follow the prompt.

Prompt: sick

       I SICK-CONTINUALLY.

1. worry
2. wrong
3. frustrated
4. careful
5. drunk
6. silly
7. mischievous
8. sad
9. depressed
10. disgusted

PLACES YOU VISITED

Alex: BEFORE I GO-THERE HOLLAND VISIT THERE FLOWER PLACE.
_____q_____
SEE^FINISH YOU?

Pat: NO. HEARD HOLLAND CL:5̈5̈⇈ FLOWER.

Alex: RIGHT. HOLLAND VERY-WET, EASY GROW. ANYWAY, 1 PLACE, DON'T-
KNOW NAME, IT SELL FLOWER++. I VERY-IMPRESSED I. I ENTER
BUILDING, SEE FLOWER ALL-OVER. COLOR LOUD. ODD, THAT TIME
DURING AUTUMN, VERY-COLD OUTSIDE. WHERE FLOWER FROM
I WONDER.

Key Structures

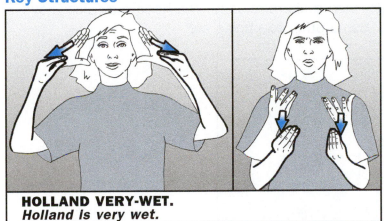

HOLLAND VERY-WET.
Holland is very wet.

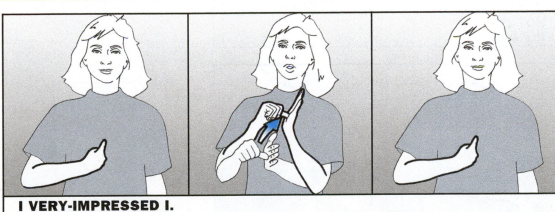

I VERY-IMPRESSED I.
I was very impressed.

20

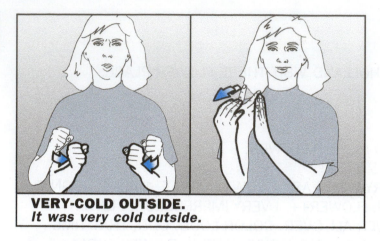

VERY-COLD OUTSIDE.
It was very cold outside.

Grammar Note

Some adjectives such as WET, IMPRESSED, and COLD in the previous sentences change their movement to show intensity. This is done by a hold at the beginning of the sign, then a sharp release. The head may also move sharply during the release. Some other examples are:

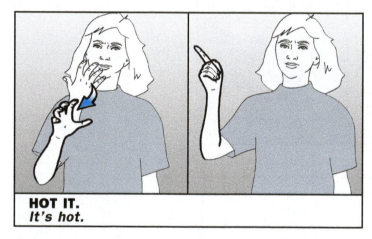

HOT IT.
It's hot.

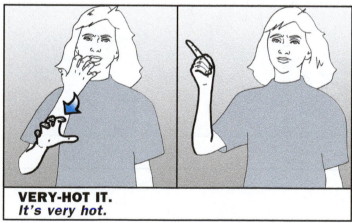

VERY-HOT IT.
It's very hot.

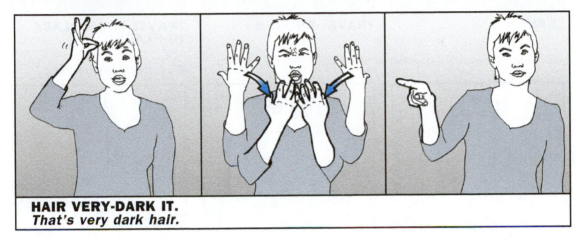

HAIR DARK IT.
That's dark hair.

HAIR VERY-DARK IT.
That's very dark hair.

Exercise 20C

Describe the following using the adjective given. Follow the prompt.

Prompt: today (very hot)

       TODAY VERY-HOT.

1. mail (very slow)
2. bed (very hard)
3. boy (very strong)
4. father (very proud)
5. president (very embarrassed)
6. food (very expensive)
7. supervisor (very strict)
8. dog (very fat)
9. runner (very fast)
10. yesterday (very cold)

20

VOCABULARY

▶ Travel

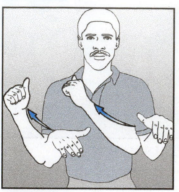

LEAVE

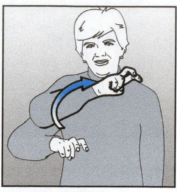

TRAVEL-AROUND

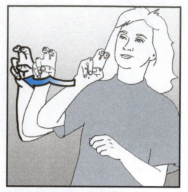

TRAVEL-FROM-PLACE TO-PLACE

▶ Noun-Verb Pairs

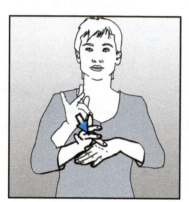

BEEN-THERE, touch

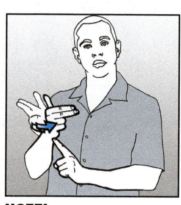

HOTEL

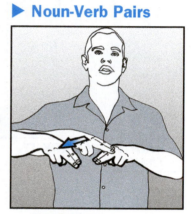

GO-BY-TRAIN, Noun: TRAIN

▶ Adjectives

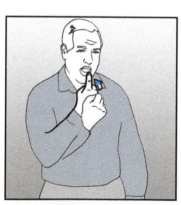

TAKE-PILL, Noun: PILL

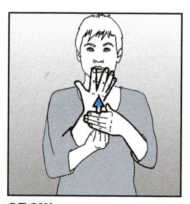

GROW, Noun: PLANT

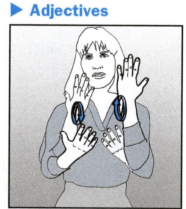

EMBARRASSED

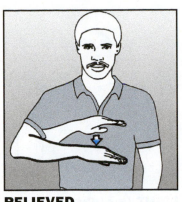

RELIEVED

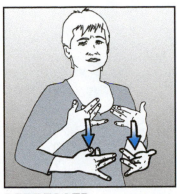

DEPRESSED

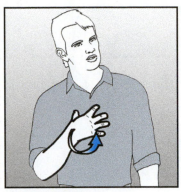

DISGUSTED

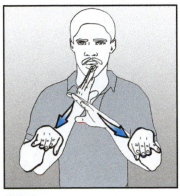

QUIET

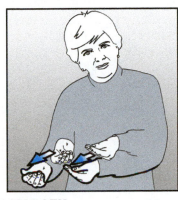

SMOOTH

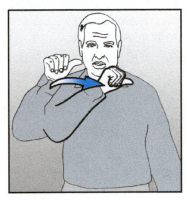

DRUNK

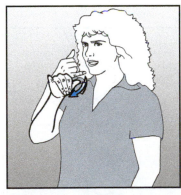

SILLY

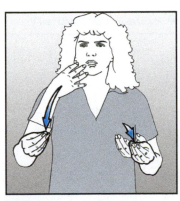

WET

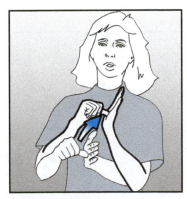

IMPRESSED

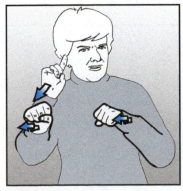

LOUD

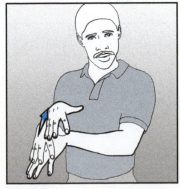

SLOW

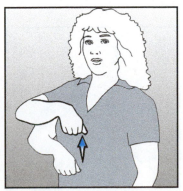

PROUD

20

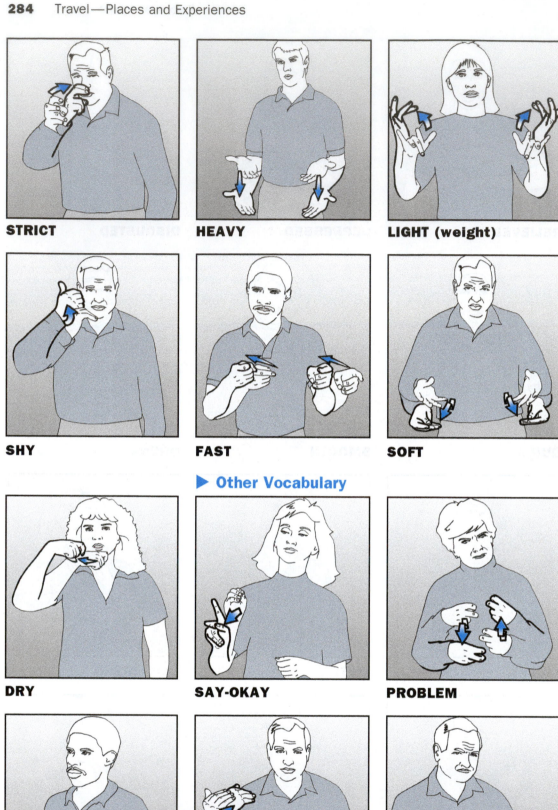

STRICT   **HEAVY**   **LIGHT (weight)**

SHY   **FAST**   **SOFT**

▶ **Other Vocabulary**

DRY   **SAY-OKAY**   **PROBLEM**

HEART   **REMIND**   **TEND-TO**

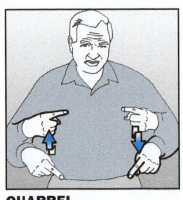

QUARREL

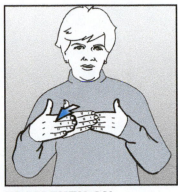

FROM-THEN-ON

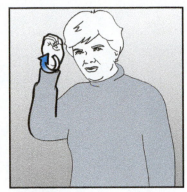

EUROPE

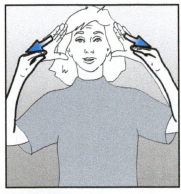

HOLLAND

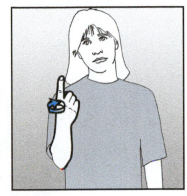

ALONE

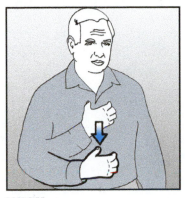

WISH

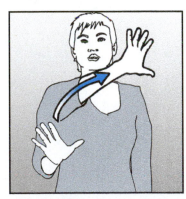

ALL-OVER

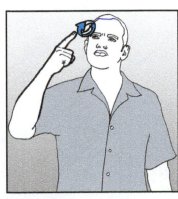

WONDER

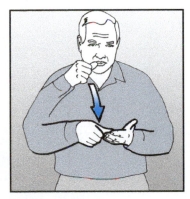

MAIL, letter

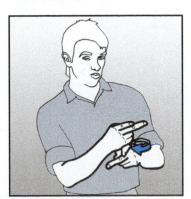

SUPERVISOR

20

UNIT 21

Occupations and Professions

In this unit, you will learn to talk about occupations and professions, including job activity and work experience.

You will learn vocabulary that can incorporate an agent suffix such as WELDER and MECHANIC.

You will learn to ask rhetorical questions and to use UNDERSTAND to precede a qualification, condition, or stipulation.

OCCUPATIONS AND PROFESSIONS

Alex: _____whq_____
YOUR WORK WHAT?

Chris: I WORK WELD I. WORK THERE BUILD SHIP SINCE TWO YEAR.

Alex: OH-I-SEE. NOT REALIZE I. THINK YOU WORK P-O, WRONG I.

Chris: NEVER P-O I. LONG-AGO I WORK CAR FIX-CAR. I SWITCH-OVER
                   __rq__   _____whq_____
SPECIALIZE WELD. WHY? SWELL MONEY. YOU WORK WHAT?

Alex: I TEACH A-S-L PLUS I WORK PAINT.
       ____whq____
Chris: PAINT WHAT?

Alex: HOUSE, BUILDING, BRIDGE, ANY.

Key Structures

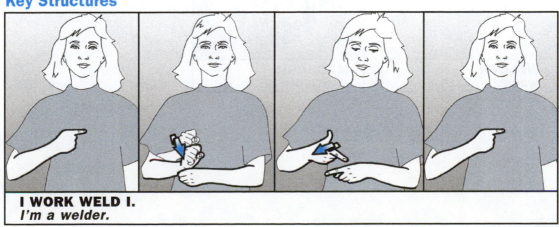

I WORK WELD I.
I'm a welder.

287

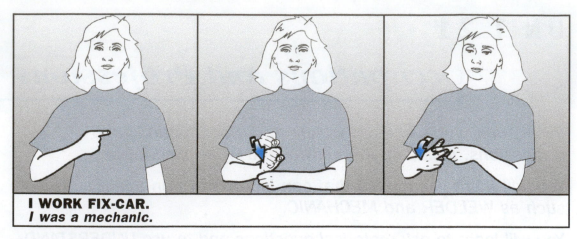

I WORK FIX-CAR.
I was a mechanic.

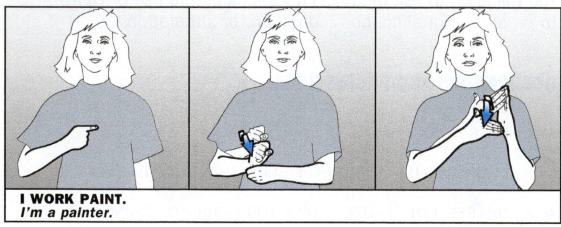

I WORK PAINT.
I'm a painter.

Grammar Note

Some signs for types of work may be accompanied by an agent suffix as in the following:

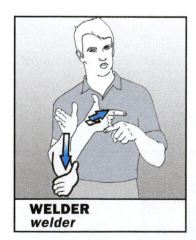

WELDER
welder

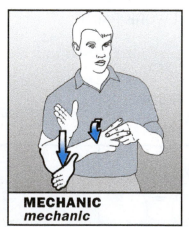

MECHANIC
mechanic

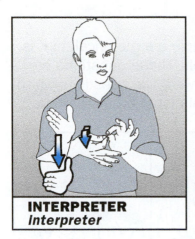

INTERPRETER
interpreter

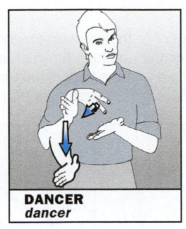

DANCER
dancer

Some signs for occupations or professions do not use the agent suffix. Some examples are:

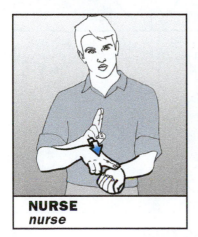

NURSE
nurse

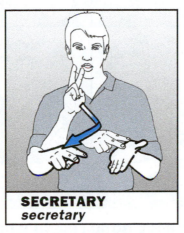

SECRETARY
secretary

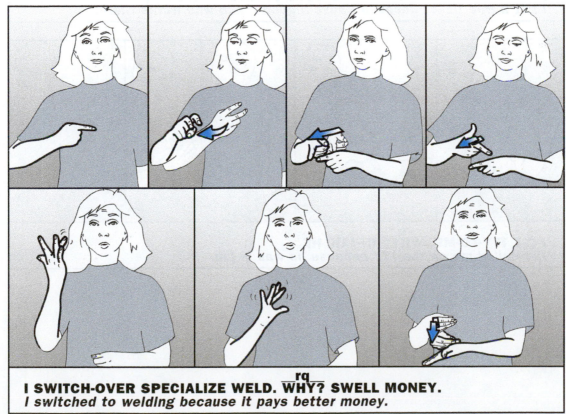

rq
I SWITCH-OVER SPECIALIZE WELD. WHY? SWELL MONEY.
I switched to welding because it pays better money.

21

Grammar Note

Some questions such as WHY? in the preceding example are rhetorical, that is, the signer intends to answer the question him/herself. These questions are made with the eyebrows raised and the head tilted forward like questions which ask for a yes/no answer. Some other examples of this type of question are:

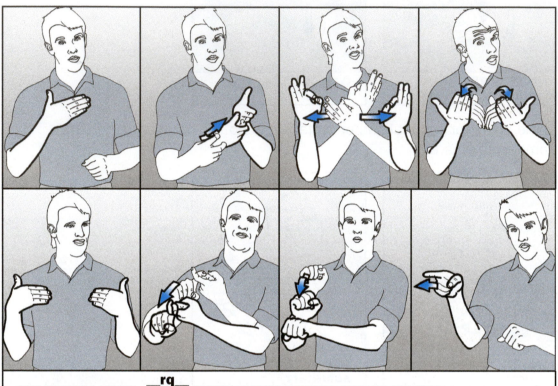

MY TICKET FREE. $\overline{\text{HOW?}}^{\text{rq}}$ HAVE GOOD-FRIEND WORK THERE.
I got a free ticket because I have a good friend who works there.

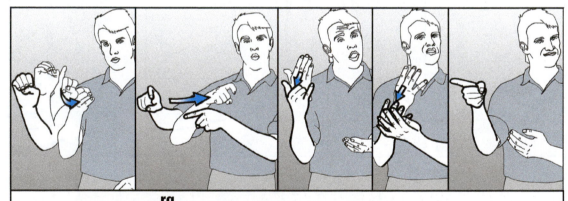

J-O-E TTY-TO-ME. $\overline{\text{WHY?}}^{\text{rq}}$ IN-JAIL HE.
Joe called me on the TTY because he was in jail.

Exercise 21A

Ask your partner if he/she is one of the following. Follow the prompt.

Prompt: welder

_____q_____
YOU WORK WELD YOU?

 1. computer programmer
 2. painter
 3. counselor
 4. printer
 5. post office worker
 6. actress
 7. secretary
 8. farmer
 9. doctor
10. waiter

Exercise 21B

Give the following reasons for why you aren't going. Follow the prompt.

Prompt: Your car was stolen.

_rq_
I NOT GO-THERE I. WHY? CAR STEAL.

 1. You have no money.
 2. You don't like to fly.
 3. You weren't invited.
 4. You don't like the cold.

Tell where you found the ring. Follow the prompt.

Prompt: under the bed

___rq___
I FIND RING. WHERE? UNDER BED.

 5. behind the door
 6. in your pocket
 7. in the grass
 8. on the shelf

21

JOB ACTIVITY

<pre>
                         _____q_____
Pat: YOU WORK B-A-N-K RIGHT?

Lisa: RIGHT.
                  _____whq_____
Pat: EXACT WORK WHAT?

Lisa: I WORK FEED COMPUTER. CHECK++, DEPOSIT++ CL:L̈-STACK, I TYPE
                                             _____t_____
         FEED. I SUPERVISOR, HAVE SUBORDINATE++ 3. PROBLEM SHOW-UP,

         I HELP SOLVE.
                 _____q_____
Pat: WORK DAY++?

Lisa: YES. I WORK 4-DAY. UNDERSTAND, 10 HOUR STRAIGHT
                 _____t_____
         LEFT 3-DAY, OFF.

Pat: OH-I-SEE. SWELL IDEA.
</pre>

Key Structures

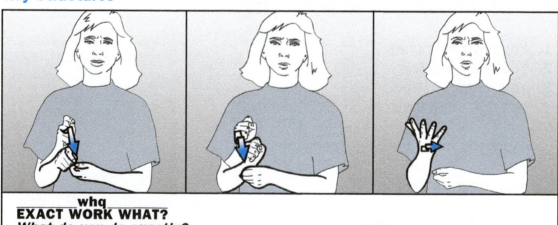

<pre>
           whq
EXACT WORK WHAT?
</pre>
What do you do exactly?

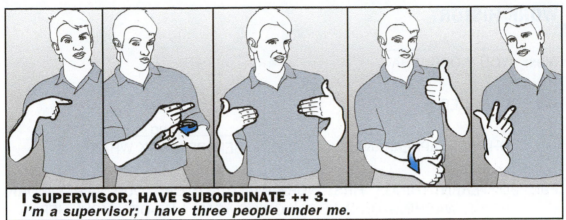

I SUPERVISOR, HAVE SUBORDINATE ++ 3.
I'm a supervisor; I have three people under me.

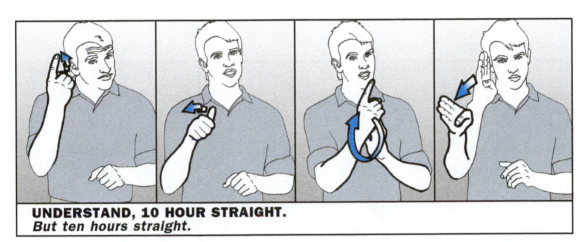

UNDERSTAND, 10 HOUR STRAIGHT.
But ten hours straight.

Note

As in the preceding sentence, a form of the sign UNDERSTAND is often used to precede a qualification, condition, or stipulation which the signer will state.

Exercise 21C

Describe the job you now have or the job you last had. Give details of what work you do (did) and what your hours are (were).

21

WORK HISTORY

```
          _____whq_____
```
Alex: YOU WORK WHAT?

Pat: I RETIRED I.

```
                                    _____whq_____
```
Alex: OH-I-SEE. APPEARANCE YOUNG YOU. BEFORE WORK WHAT?

Pat: DIFFERENT-THINGS. FIRST WORK PAINT. NOT LIKE, QUIT. APPLY WORK
        PRINT, WASHINGTON P-O-S-T. WORK 6 YEAR, LAID-OFF, MOVE-HERE
        L-A. LOOK #JOB, CAN'T FIND, I GET-REGULARLY. LATER L-A T-I-M-E-S
        HIRE-ME. WORK 30 YEAR, SINCE EVERY-NIGHT. NOW RETIRED.

Key Structures

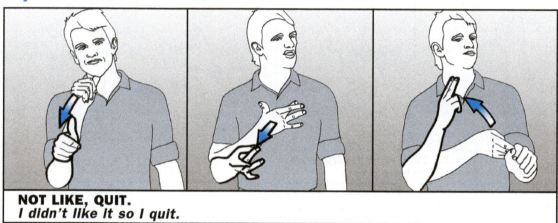

NOT LIKE, QUIT.
I didn't like it so I quit.

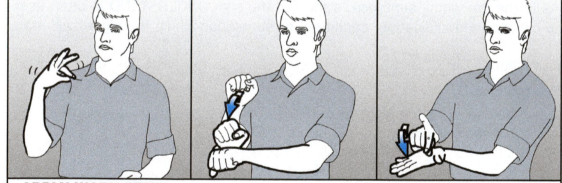

APPLY WORK PRINT.
I applied for work as a printer.

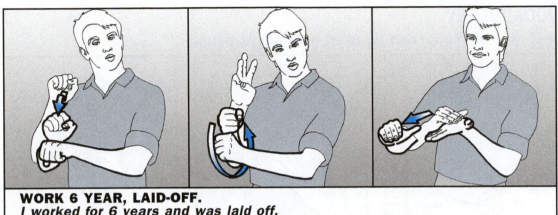

WORK 6 YEAR, LAID-OFF.
I worked for 6 years and was laid off.

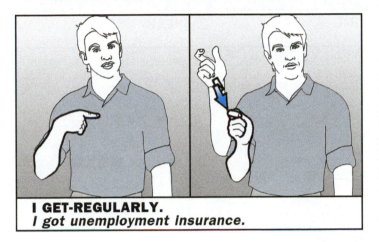

I GET-REGULARLY.
I got unemployment Insurance.

Note

The sign GET-REGULARLY in the context above means to get unemployment payments or any form of public assistance, including Social Security payments. It also can mean getting regular payments from a pension or an annuity.

In addition, GET-REGULARLY can mean to subscribe or receive something on a regular basis like a magazine or newsletter.

Exercise 21D

Make up a work history that includes at least three past jobs. Give this work history, name the jobs, where they were, tell a little about each job and why you left, and tell about your present job or the job you hope to get in the future.

21

VOCABULARY

▶ **Types of Work (can be used with agent suffix)**

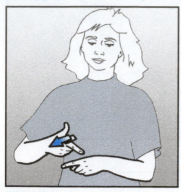

WELD

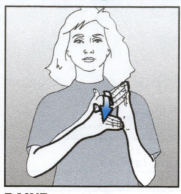

PAINT

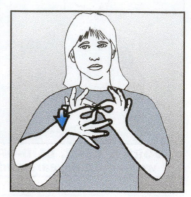

INTERPRET

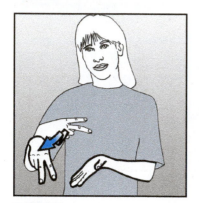

DANCE

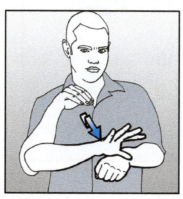

COUNSEL

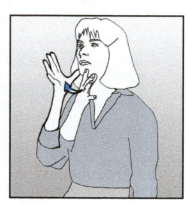

FARM

▶ **Occupations and Professions
(not used with agent suffix)**

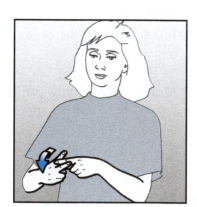

FIX-CAR

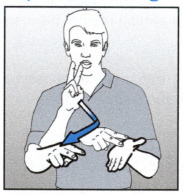

SECRETARY

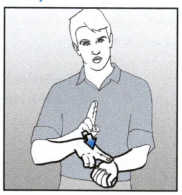

NURSE

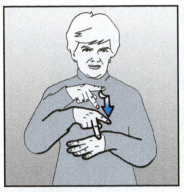

PRINCIPAL

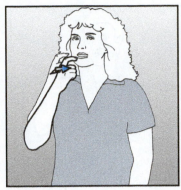

DENTIST

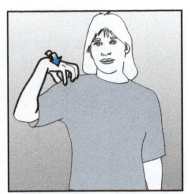

BOSS

▶ **Personnel Matters**

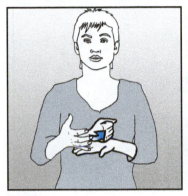

EARN

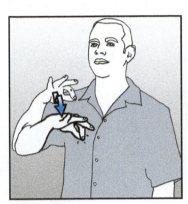

BENEFITS

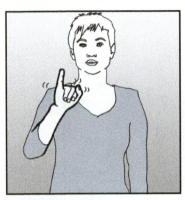

INSURANCE

▶ **Clergy**

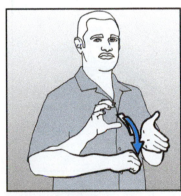

DEDUCTIONS

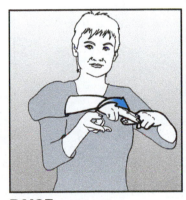

RAISE

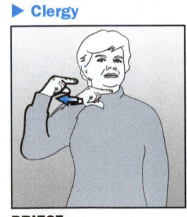

PRIEST

▶ **Other Vocabulary**

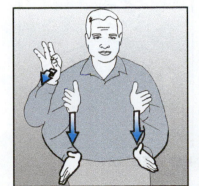

PREACHER, pastor

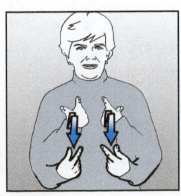

RABBI

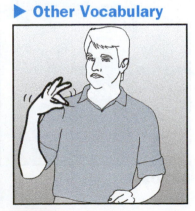

APPLY

21

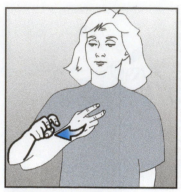

SWITCH-OVER

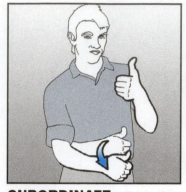

SUBORDINATE

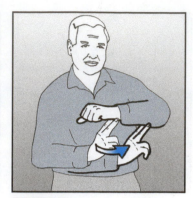

BRIDGE

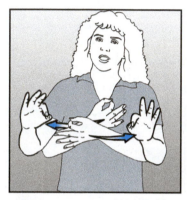

FREE

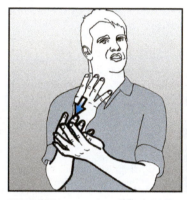

IN-JAIL

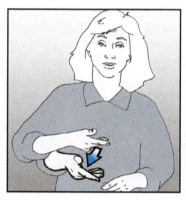

INVITE

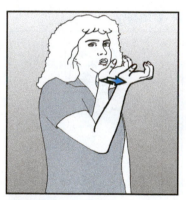

GRASS

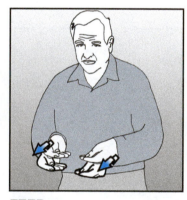

FEED

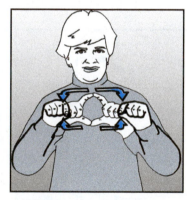

CHECK

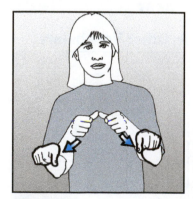

DEPOSIT

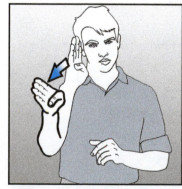

STRAIGHT

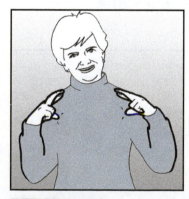

RETIRED, off

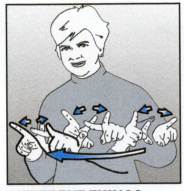

DIFFERENT-THINGS

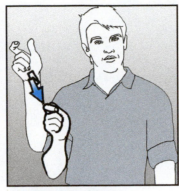

GET-REGULARLY

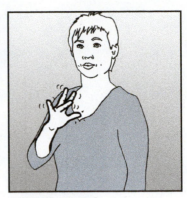

SWELL, cool

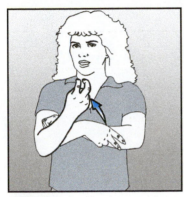

STEAL

21

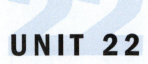

UNIT 22

The Body, Health, and Emergencies

In this unit you will learn to talk about your health, physical conditioning, and about emergencies.

You will learn about using the body as a pronoun and how PAIN can be moved to different locations on the body to indicate different sources of pain.

In a culture note, you will learn about some of the ways Deaf people communicate with non-signers.

PHYSICAL CONDITIONING

Chris: WOW! APPEARANCE GOOD YOU. EXERCISE YOU?
                                        _____q_____

Lisa: YES. EVERYDAY I RUN APPROXIMATELY 3, 4 M-I-L-E-S.

Chris: IMPRESSED I. I GO-THERE-REPEATEDLY S-P-A LIFT-WEIGHTS I.

            _____q_____

Lisa: YOU WEIGH CL:11-LEGS-LIFT-UP-AND-DOWN YOU?

Chris: YES. PLUS WEIGH CL:SS-PUT-ON-SHOULDERS CL:∧-BEND-KNEES-UP-AND-DOWN.

            _____q_____

Lisa: WANT YOU ACCOMPANY-ME RUN?

Chris: NO. RUN, BORED I.

22

Key Structures

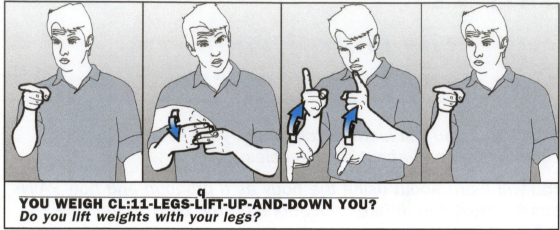

q
YOU WEIGH CL:11-LEGS-LIFT-UP-AND-DOWN YOU?
Do you lift weights with your legs?

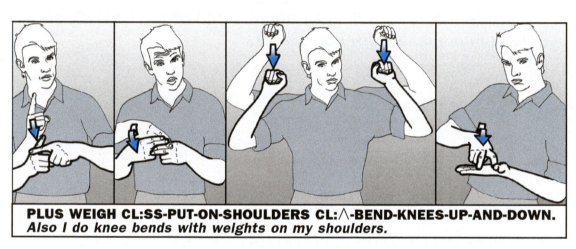

PLUS WEIGH CL:SS-PUT-ON-SHOULDERS CL:∧-BEND-KNEES-UP-AND-DOWN.
Also I do knee bends with weights on my shoulders.

Grammar Note

In the preceding sentence, the body (or limbs) of the signer is used as a pronoun to indicate what is done with the weights.

Exercise 22A

Describe five types of physical exercise to your partner.

HEALTH AND HEALTH PROBLEMS

Lisa: __whq__
HEAR YOU HOSPITAL. HAPPEN?

Alex: YES. I ALMOST HEART-ATTACK I. NOT BAD. I FINE I.

Lisa: _____whq_____
OH-I-SEE. DON'T-KNOW I. HOW HAPPEN?

Alex: SINCE I PRESSURE, NONE EXERCISE, EAT-CONTINUALLY. I WORK,
FEEL PAIN-IN-CHEST 2-DAY, 3-DAY. DECIDE GO-THERE DOCTOR.
DOCTOR LOOK-OVER TAKE-BLOOD-PRESSURE. WOW! HIGH.
IMMEDIATELY CARRY-ME HOSPITAL. MUST CL:∧-LIE-IN-BED, TAKE-PILL-
REPEATEDLY, STAY 1-WEEK. FINISH GO-THERE HOME, NONE WORK
2-MONTH. WELL NOW, BLOOD-PRESSURE NORMAL.

Key Structures

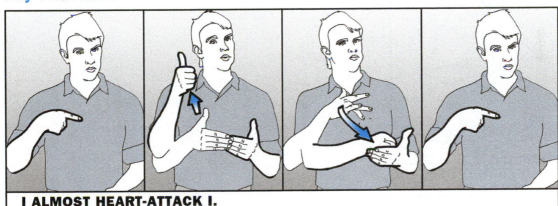

I ALMOST HEART-ATTACK I.
I almost had a heart attack.

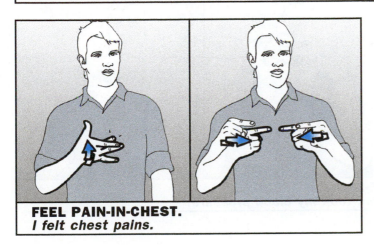

FEEL PAIN-IN-CHEST.
I felt chest pains.

22

Note

The sign PAIN can change location on the body to indicate different sources of pain as in the following examples:

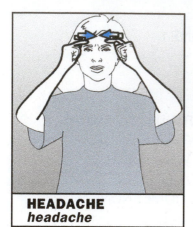

HEADACHE
headache

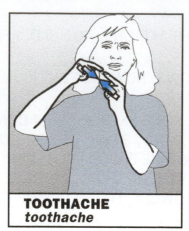

TOOTHACHE
toothache

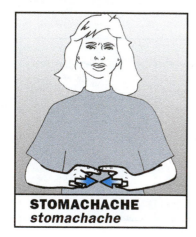

STOMACHACHE
stomachache

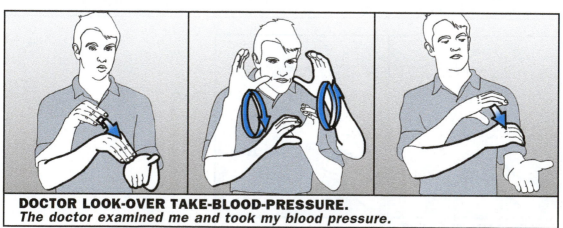

DOCTOR LOOK-OVER TAKE-BLOOD-PRESSURE.
The doctor examined me and took my blood pressure.

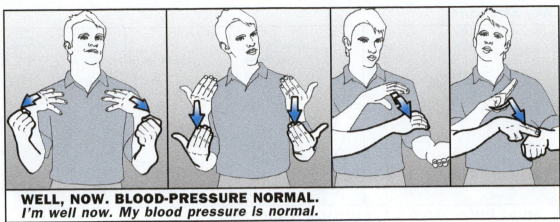

WELL, NOW. BLOOD-PRESSURE NORMAL.
I'm well now. My blood pressure is normal.

Exercise 22B

Describe the symptoms of a recent illness you or someone you know experienced. Describe what happened and how the illness was treated. Include several symptoms.

EMERGENCIES

Alex: MAN CL:∧-FALL-DOWN. SEEM SICK. MUST PHONE-TO 9-1-1, SUMMON AMBULANCE.

Chris: ASK-HER WOMAN, CAN HEAR SHE.

Alex: YOU GO-THERE COVER, KEEP WARM.

(later)

     _____q_____ _____q_____
Chris: SUCCEED? AMBULANCE COME-HERE?

Alex: YES. I WRITE CL:B-SHOW-TO WOMAN. UNDERSTAND, PHONE-TO. SHOULD ARRIVE 5-MINUTE.

         _____q_____
Chris: SEEM HE BREATHE O-K. WONDER HE FAINT?

Alex: DON'T-KNOW I. I EXPERIENCE BEFORE NEVER I.

22

Key Structures

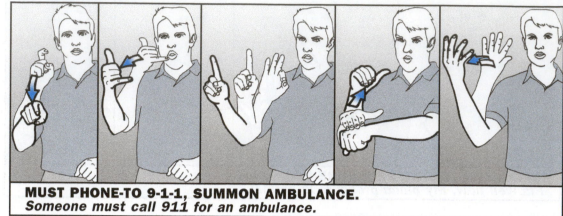

MUST PHONE-TO 9-1-1, SUMMON AMBULANCE.
Someone must call 911 for an ambulance.

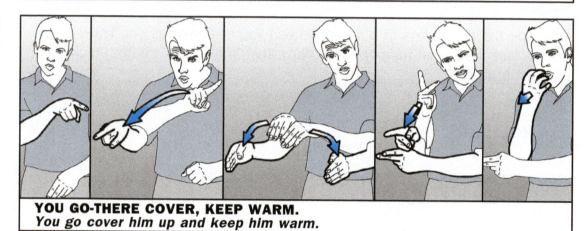

YOU GO-THERE COVER, KEEP WARM.
You go cover him up and keep him warm.

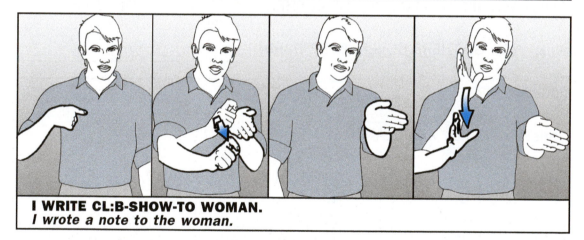

I WRITE CL:B-SHOW-TO WOMAN.
I wrote a note to the woman.

Culture Note

The interaction between the Deaf person and the woman to whom he wrote the note asking her to call an ambulance in the preceding sentence, is an example of one way that Deaf people communicate with non-signers. There are other ways of communicating including the use of gesture, speech and hearing, or lipreading. The individual's choice of strategies for communicating with non-signers is usually based on experience of what works best in interactions with non-signers.

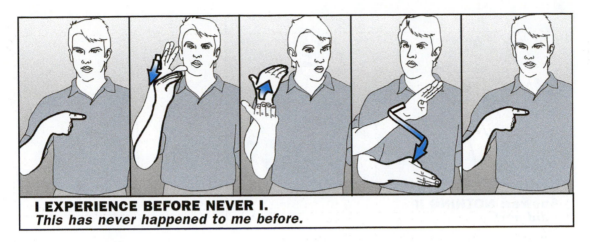

I EXPERIENCE BEFORE NEVER I.
This has never happened to me before.

Grammar Note

In the preceding sentence, NEVER is used as a negative. NEVER and NOTHING are also used as denials as in the following:

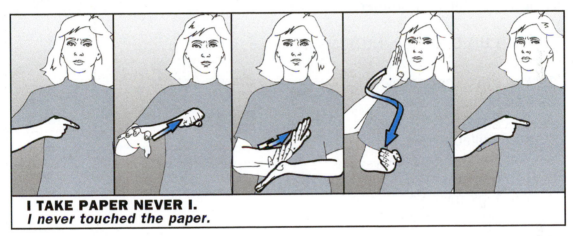

I TAKE PAPER NEVER I.
I never touched the paper.

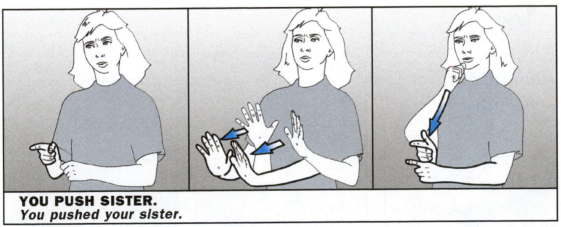

YOU PUSH SISTER.
You pushed your sister.

22

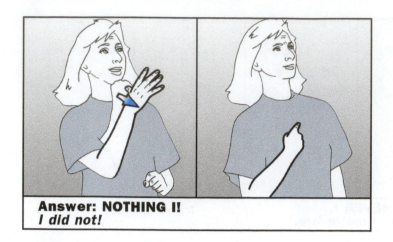

Answer: NOTHING I!
I did not!

Exercise 22C

Deny the following accusations. Follow the prompt.

Prompt: You hit your brother.

I HIT BROTHER, NOTHING I.

1. You stole the money.
2. You broke a glass.
3. You gossip.
4. You spilled water.
5. You've been smoking.
6. You helped her.
7. You took my bike.
8. You ate my cookie.
9. You're mocking me.
10. You lied.

VOCABULARY

▶ The Body

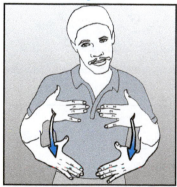

BODY, health

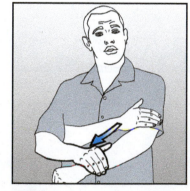

ARM

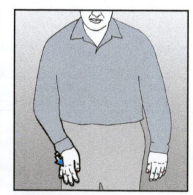

LEG

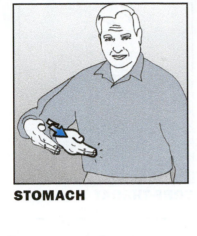

STOMACH

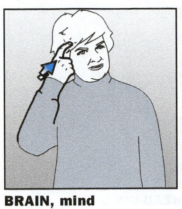

BRAIN, mind

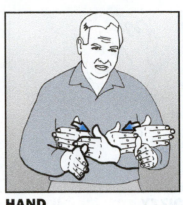

HAND

▶ **Health**

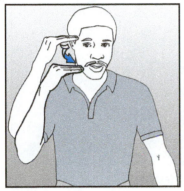

HEAD

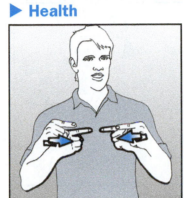

PAIN, hurt

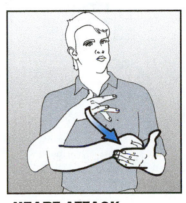

HEART-ATTACK

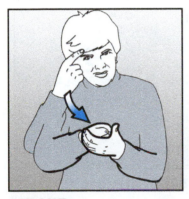

STROKE

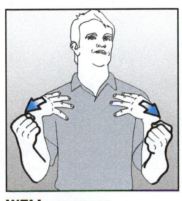

WELL, recover

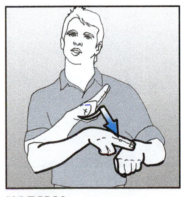

NORMAL

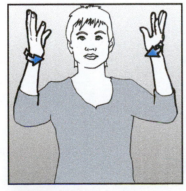

AMBULANCE

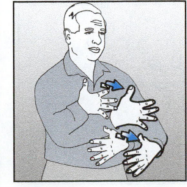

BREATHE

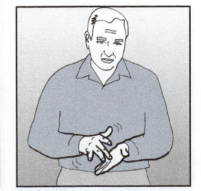

MEDICINE

22

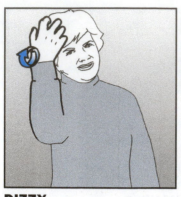

DIZZY

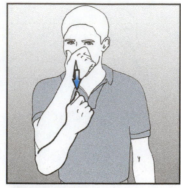

HEAD-COLD

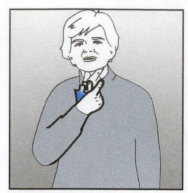

SORE-THROAT

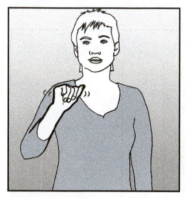

ARTHRITIS

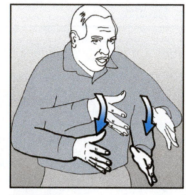

VOMIT

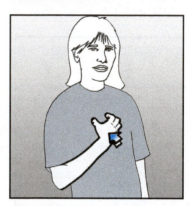

COUGH

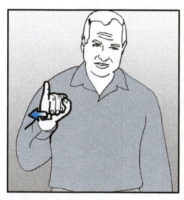

INFECTION

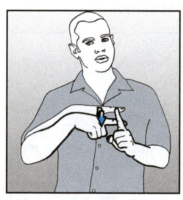

TEMPERATURE, fever

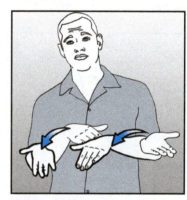

DEAD, die, death

▶ **Noun-Verb Pairs**

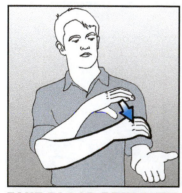

**TAKE-BLOOD-PRESSURE,
Noun: BLOOD-PRESSURE**

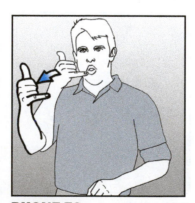

**PHONE-TO,
Noun: TELEPHONE**

▶ **Other Vocabulary**

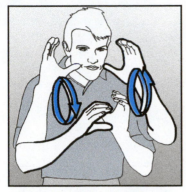

LOOK-OVER, examine

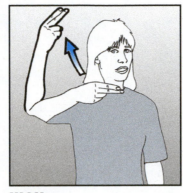

HIGH

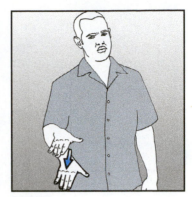

LOW

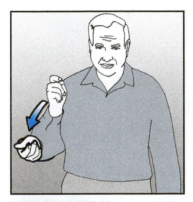

IMMEDIATELY, fast, quick

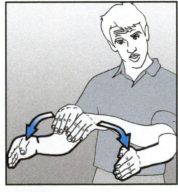

COVER

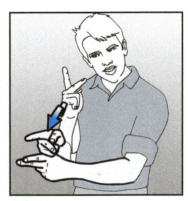

KEEP

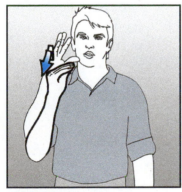

EXPERIENCE

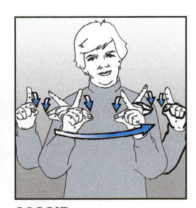

GOSSIP

22

UNIT 23

Current Events

In this unit, you will learn to talk about current events, topics, and issues.

You will learn how to relate an event that occurs several times in different places.

You will learn about using sentences that have a topic clause.

And you will learn about using WORSE in a way that can actually mean something is better.

RECENT NEWS

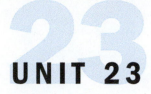

```
            _____q_____
Alex    HEAR YOU?

        _whq_
Pat:    WHAT?


Alex:   EARTH+QUAKE IN CALIFORNIA NEAR L-A. BUILDING CRACK,
        CL:BB-ROOF-FALL-IN++.

        _____whq_____ _____whq_____
Pat:    HOW KNOW YOU? WHEN HAPPEN?


Alex    MORNING. SEE T-V N-E-W-S RECENT.

        _____whq_____
Pat:    EXACT WHERE?


Alex:   SEEM S-E APPROXIMATELY.


Pat:    SON LIVE L-A. SHOULD TTY-TO CHECK.
```

Key Structures

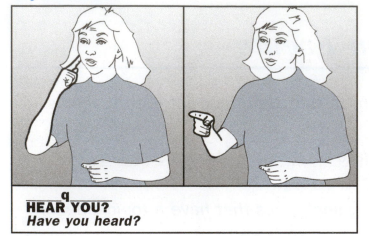

_____q
HEAR YOU?
Have you heard?

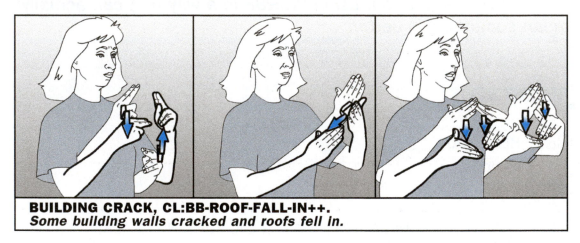

BUILDING CRACK, CL:BB-ROOF-FALL-IN++.
Some building walls cracked and roofs fell in.

Grammar Note

In CL:BB-ROOF-FALL-IN++ above, the event is shown to have occured several times in several places by reduplicating the sign with a slight shift in the location of the sign. Some other examples of this are:

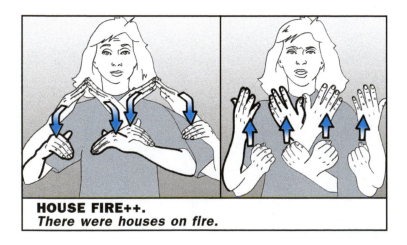

HOUSE FIRE++.
There were houses on fire.

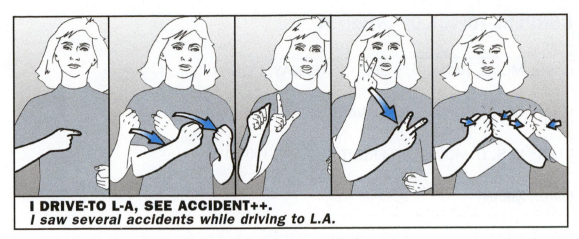

I DRIVE-TO L-A, SEE ACCIDENT++.
I saw several accidents while driving to L.A.

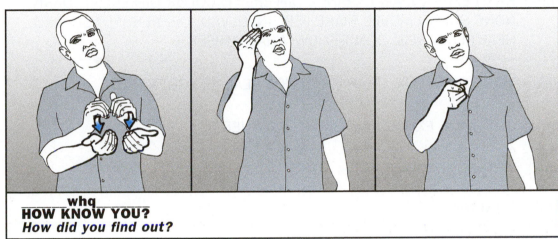

whq
HOW KNOW YOU?
How did you find out?

Exercise 23A

Describe an event from yesterday's news in detail. Your partner will ask questions for clarification.

Exercise 23B

Tell your partner that the following events happened in several places. Follow the prompt.

Prompt: Several people slipped on ice in the street.

STREET FREEZE, PEOPLE CL:∧-FALL-DOWN++.

1. Several trees fell down.
2. Several buildings were razed.
3. Several people were laid up (became sick).
4. Several cars broke down.
5. Several walls were cracked.
6. Several bicycles fell over in the wind.

23

CURRENT TOPICS OF INTEREST

_____t_____
Chris: MOVIE TWO-OF-US SEE YESTERDAY, I LIKE I.

Lisa: SAME-AS-YOU LIKE I. WANT SEE AGAIN I.

Chris: YES. IT MOVIE DIFFERENT IT, HARD EXPLAIN.
        __whq__
Lisa: MEAN?

Chris: HARD EXPLAIN. APPEARANCE DIFFERENT, COLOR DIFFERENT, DARK.
        NONE SUN IN MOVIE. MAKE FEEL INVOLVED. DEPRESSED, SCARED,
        HEART-LURCHES. DON'T-KNOW WHAT HAPPEN.

Lisa: TRUE, BUT SOME CHARACTER NOT REAL, EXAGGERATED.

Chris: BUT SOME EXACT, LIKE SMALL BROTHER.

Lisa: YES. GOOD MOVIE.

Key Structures

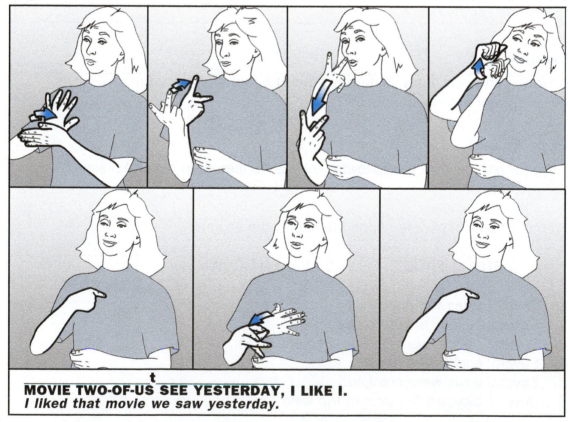

t
MOVIE TWO-OF-US SEE YESTERDAY, I LIKE I.
I liked that movie we saw yesterday.

Grammar Note

In discussing events or topics, a clause can be used as the topic of a sentence and a comment made about the topic as in the following examples:

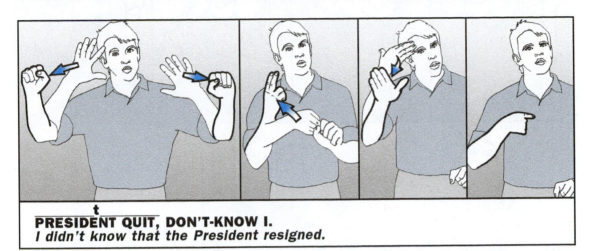

t
PRESIDENT QUIT, DON'T-KNOW I.
I didn't know that the President resigned.

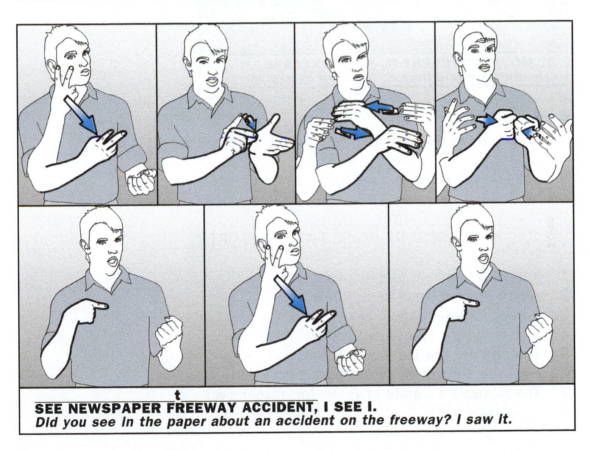

t
SEE NEWSPAPER FREEWAY ACCIDENT, I SEE I.
Did you see in the paper about an accident on the freeway? I saw it.

23

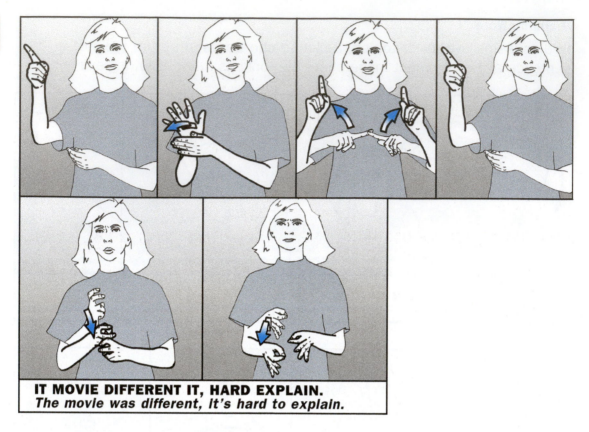

IT MOVIE DIFFERENT IT, HARD EXPLAIN.
The movie was different, it's hard to explain.

Exercise 23C

Comment on the following topics. Follow the prompt.

Prompt: He proposed to increase taxes. (support)

<u>   t   </u>
HE SUGGEST INCREASE T-A-X, I SUPPORT I.

1. Yesterday we lost. (depressed)
2. A new teacher was hired. (thrilled)
3. A new freeway opened. (wide)
4. I loaned you a new book. (good?)
5. The play we saw last night. (long)
6. I saw the President's speech. (did not like)
7. The restaurant we ate at yesterday. (expensive)

CURRENT ISSUES

        ———————t———————

Lisa: WORSE PROBLEM, PEOPLE POOR. ALL COUNTRY HAVE. I

        UNDERSTAND POOR COUNTRY HAVE POOR PEOPLE. WORSE, HERE

        U-S HAVE POOR PEOPLE. NOT UNDERSTAND.

Pat: RIGHT. HERE U-S MANY PEOPLE HAVE MONEY.

Lisa: MANY PEOPLE POOR, NOT THEIR FAULT. SOME CAN'T WORK, HAVE

        HEALTH PROBLEM. SOME CAN WORK BUT NOT HAVE SKILL. MANY

        OLD CAN'T WORK. GOVERNMENT SUPPORT, BUT NOT ENOUGH.
        whq
        #DO?

        ———————q———————
Pat: YOU-ASK-ME? SAME-AS-YOU DON'T-KNOW ANSWER I.

Key Structures

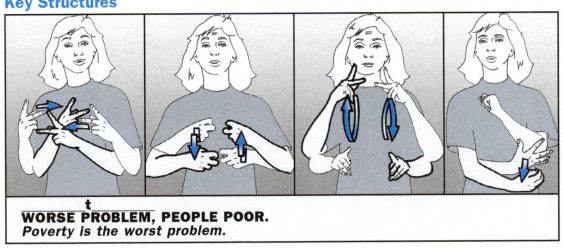

        ——————t——————
WORSE PROBLEM, PEOPLE POOR.
Poverty is the worst problem.

23

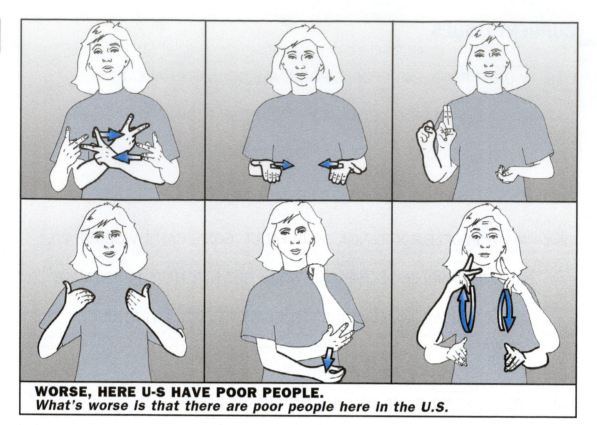

WORSE, HERE U-S HAVE POOR PEOPLE.
What's worse is that there are poor people here in the U.S.

Note

In the preceding sentence, WORSE is used to indicate that something is worse than in the previous statement. However, WORSE can be used to indicate that something is better, as in the following example:

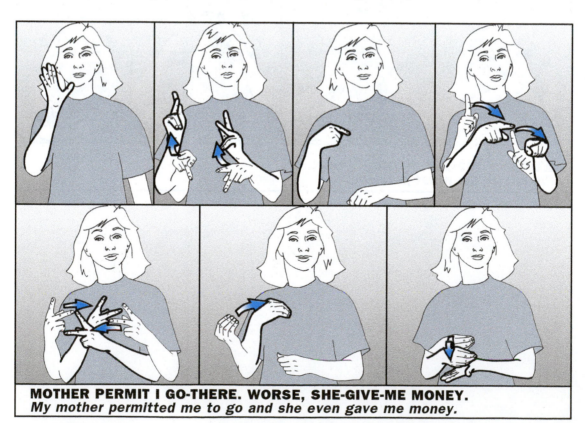

MOTHER PERMIT I GO-THERE. WORSE, SHE-GIVE-ME MONEY.
My mother permitted me to go and she even gave me money.

Exercise 23D
Discuss briefly an issue that is currently in the news. You don't have to give your opinion, just tell about the issue.

VOCABULARY

▶ **Politics**

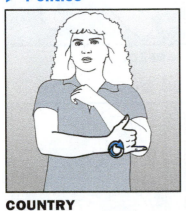

COUNTRY

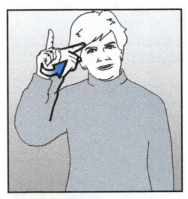

NATION

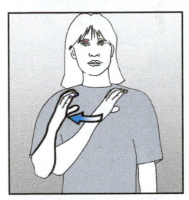

GOVERNMENT

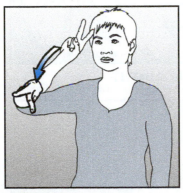

VICE-PRESIDENT

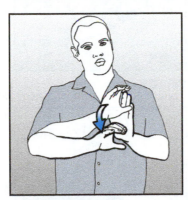

CONSTITUTION

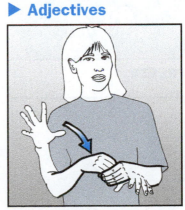

CONGRESS

▶ **Adjectives**

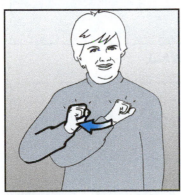

SENATE

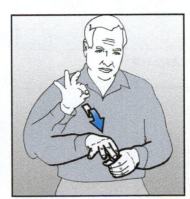

VOTE

INVOLVED

23

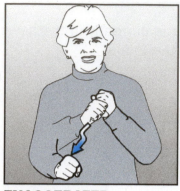

SCARED

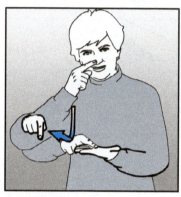

EXAGGERATED

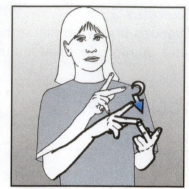

PERFECT

▶ **Other Vocabulary**

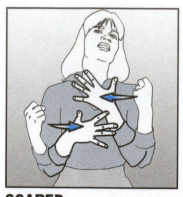

CRACK

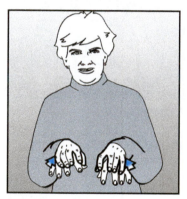

CHECK

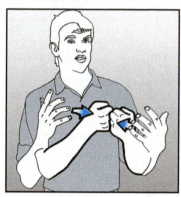

ACCIDENT

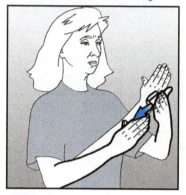

FREEZE

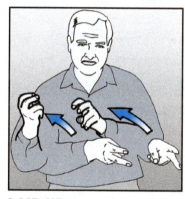

LAID-UP

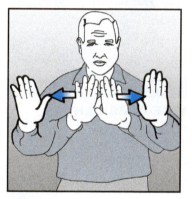

WALL

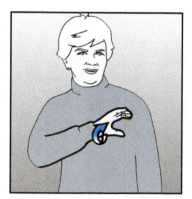

CHARACTER

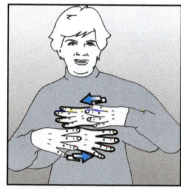

FREEWAY

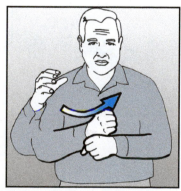

WIN

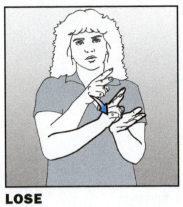

LOSE

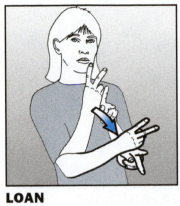

LOAN

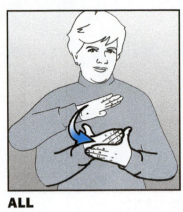

ALL

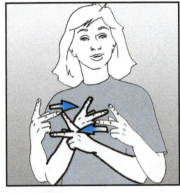

WORSE

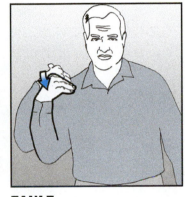

FAULT

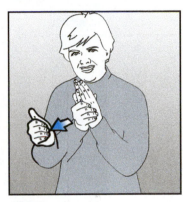

SKILL

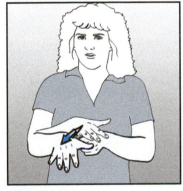

ENOUGH

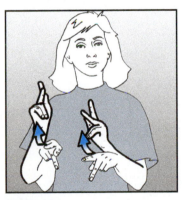

PERMIT

23

UNIT 24

How Things Are Done

In this unit, you will talk about how things are done and how to indicate different measurements.

You will learn two classifiers which show the manner in which something flows. And you will learn a classifier that is used to indicate the distance from one point to another.

And you will learn to use HOW-MUCH to ask about measurements.

A PROCESS

Lisa: SOMETHING WRONG. MACHINE NOT WORK. #DO?
                                                     whq

         __whq__
Alex: HAPPEN?

Lisa: PAPER CL:44⇉-RUNS-THROUGH-MACHINE FINE. . .CL:44⇉-STOP.

Alex: LET-ME-SEE. OH-I-SEE. LIGHT-ON MEAN PAPER STUCK INSIDE. MUST CL:S-OPEN-DOOR-ON-MACHINE, CL:S-PULL-OUT-TRAY, TAKE PAPER.

Lisa: YOU TAKE PAPER. I AWKWARD I.

Alex: NO. MUST LEARN. YOURSELF TAKE.

Key Structures

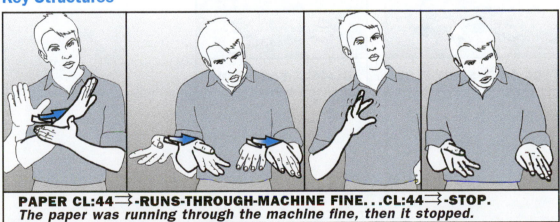

PAPER CL:44⇉-RUNS-THROUGH-MACHINE FINE. . .CL:44⇉-STOP.
The paper was running through the machine fine, then it stopped.

24

Grammar Note

In the preceding sentence the classifier predicate, CL:44⇉, shows the manner in which something flows. Some other examples of the use of CL:44⇉ and CL:4↓ are shown below:

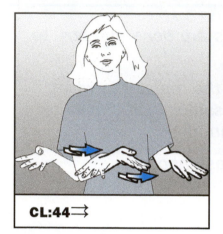

CL:44⇉

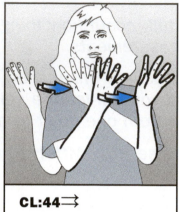

CL:44⇉

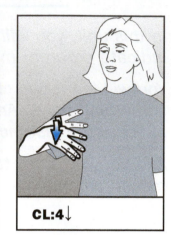

CL:4↓

indicates objects moving by, such as paper through a copying machine, newspapers through a press, or cars through an assembly line

indicates people filing past

indicates a flow of liquid such as toner pouring from a bottle, or water from a tap

With both CL:44⇉ and CL:4↓, the movement can be changed to show the speed of the flow. A smaller, more repeated movement shows a faster flow. Compare the following:

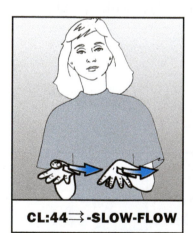

CL:44⇉-SLOW-FLOW

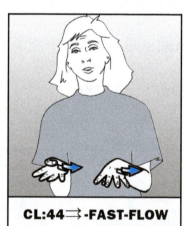

CL:44⇉-FAST-FLOW

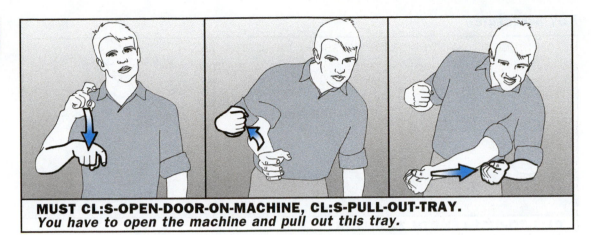

MUST CL:S-OPEN-DOOR-ON-MACHINE, CL:S-PULL-OUT-TRAY.
You have to open the machine and pull out this tray.

Exercise 24A

Describe how something works. Some examples from which you may choose:

1. changing the oil in a car
2. fixing a leaky faucet
3. putting in a sprinkler system for a garden
4. unclogging a stopped-up drain
5. changing the ribbon on a typewriter or printer
6. mixing paint to get the right color
7. running an offset printer
8. doing a chemistry experiment
9. bottling a beverage on an assembly line
10. making jelly or jam

WIDTH, LENGTH, AND HEIGHT

Chris: I WANT SHOW-YOU TABLE MYSELF MAKE.

            _____q_____
Pat: YOU MAKE DINING TABLE?

Chris: YES. I FINISH MAKE CL:BB-TABLE-TOP. CL:1-TO-CL:1-LENGTH
        72 I-N-C-H. CL:1-TO-CL:1-WIDTH 36 I-N-C-H.

        _____whq_____
Pat: HOW MAKE IT?

Chris: WOOD CL:B-PUT-AGAINST-CL:B++. NOW CL:CC-LEGS I MEASURE
        CUT-OFF. I WANT TABLE CL:1-TO-CL:1-HEIGHT 30 I-N-C-H.

        _____whq_____
Pat: HOW KNOW MEASURE YOU?

Chris: OTHER TABLE, I COPY.

24

Key Structures

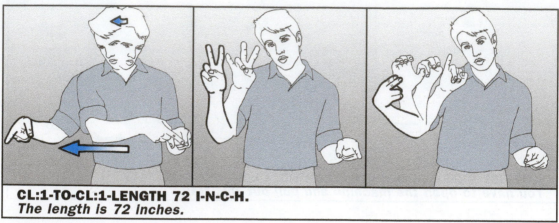

CL:1-TO-CL:1-LENGTH 72 I-N-C-H.
The length is 72 inches.

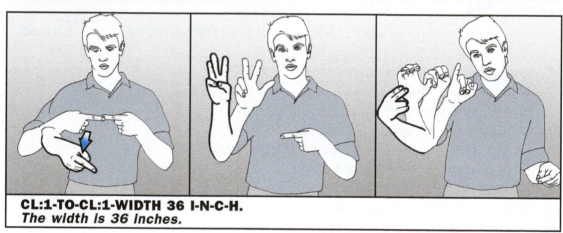

CL:1-TO-CL:1-WIDTH 36 I-N-C-H.
The width is 36 inches.

Grammar Note

The distance from one point to another can be indicated by using the classifier CL:1-TO-CL:1. Note that when stating the measurements, one hand is anchored at the starting point. Some other widths, lengths, and heights which can be indicated by CL:1-TO-CL:1 are:

    the width of a road
    the distance from one location to another or one object to another
    the height of a wall
    the length of a rope
    the distance from San Diego to Los Angeles

Exercise 24B

Indicate the width, length, height or distance of the following:

1. the measurements of the floor of the room you are in
2. the height of the ceiling of the room you are in
3. the width and height of this book
4. the distance between your home and the place where you are taking your class
5. the distance from New York to Los Angeles
6. the width and height of the blackboard in your classroom
7. the width of a road
8. the length of a rope

MEASUREMENTS AND WEIGHT

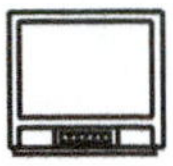

                                               __whq__
Lisa: WOW! CHRISTMAS BOX++ MANY. IT BOX, INSIDE?

Chris: SECRET. NO, NOT SECRET. INSIDE HAVE NEW T-V.

                                              ____whq____
Lisa: WOW! MEASURE CL:1-TO-CL:1-DIAGONAL HOW-MUCH?

Chris: 19 I-N-C-H.

                        __whq__
Lisa: NICE. IT BOX, INSIDE?

Chris: IT CANDY FOR GRANDMOTHER.

                          _____whq_____
Lisa: WOW! HEAVY. WEIGH HOW-MUCH IT?

Chris: 3 L-B.

                    _____whq_____
Lisa: GRANDMOTHER WEIGH HOW-MUCH?

Chris: SILLY FINISH.

24

Key Structures

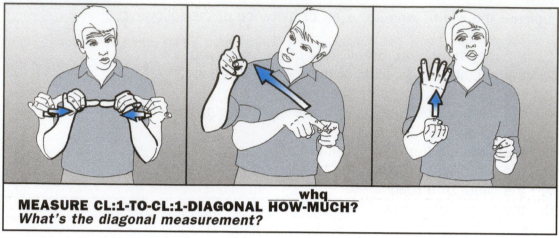

MEASURE CL:1-TO-CL:1-DIAGONAL $\overline{\text{HOW-MUCH?}}^{\text{whq}}$
What's the diagonal measurement?

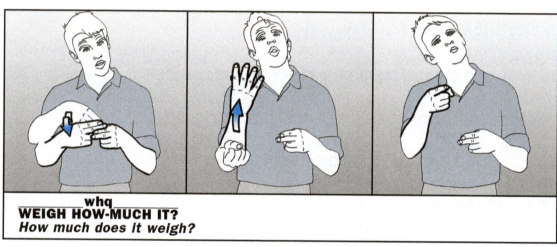

$\overline{\text{WEIGH HOW-MUCH IT?}}^{\text{whq}}$
How much does it weigh?

Grammar Note

HOW-MUCH is used to ask about measurements, height, and weight. Note that when asking about measurements one hand is anchored at the starting point while the other signs HOW-MUCH.

You may ask about height and weight without using HOW-MUCH as in the following examples:

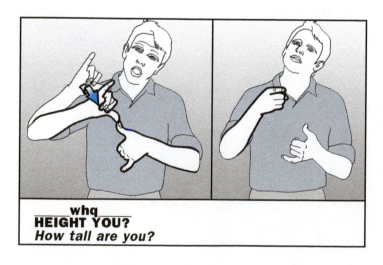

$\overline{\text{HEIGHT YOU?}}^{\text{whq}}$
How tall are you?

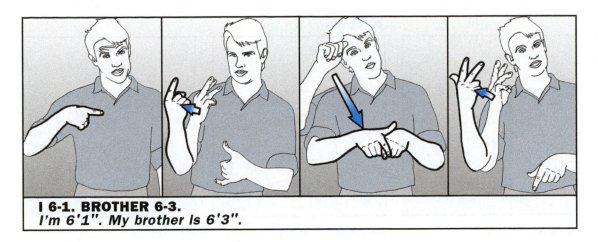

I 6-1. BROTHER 6-3.
I'm 6'1". My brother is 6'3".

Exercise 24C

Ask for the measurements of all the items in Exercise 24B.

Also, ask the height and weight of several of your classmates. Your classmates may give true or false answers to your questions. If they give false answers, you say SILLY FINISH.

VOCABULARY

▶ **Materials**

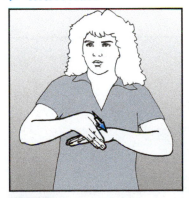

WOOD

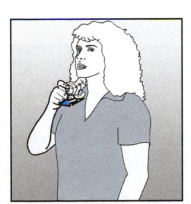

METAL

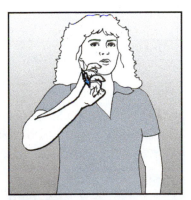

RUBBER

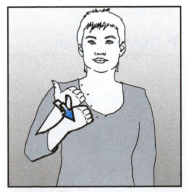

LEATHER

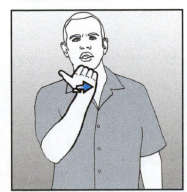

CLOTH

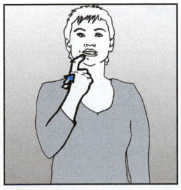

GLASS

24

▶ Tools

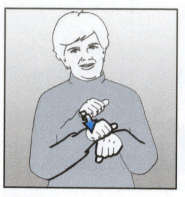

ROCK

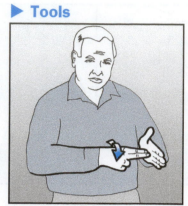

SCREWDRIVER

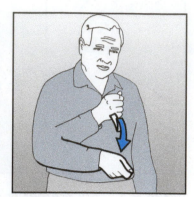

HAMMER

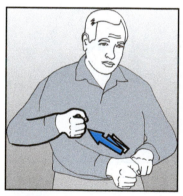

WRENCH

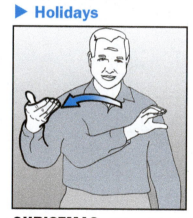

PLIERS

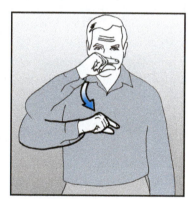

DRILL

▶ Holidays

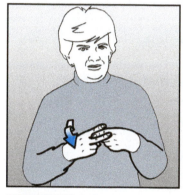

SAW

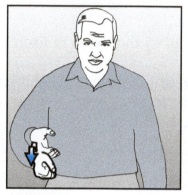

CHRISTMAS

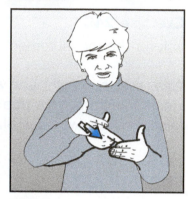

THANKSGIVING

▶ Question Sign

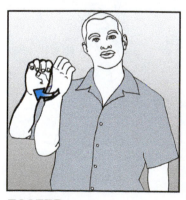

EASTER

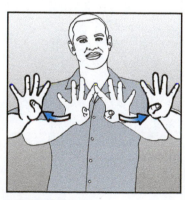

HANUKKAH

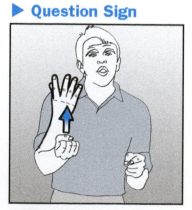

HOW-MUCH

▶ **Other Vocabulary**

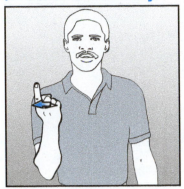

SOMETHING

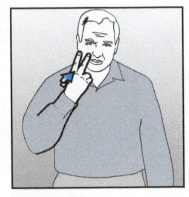

LET'S-SEE

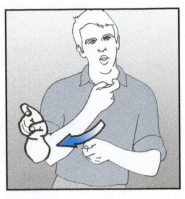

RUIN

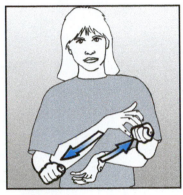

DESTROY

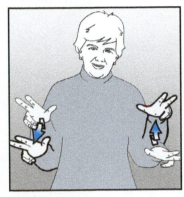

AWKWARD

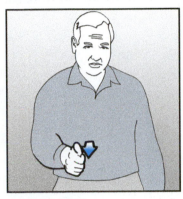

YOURSELF

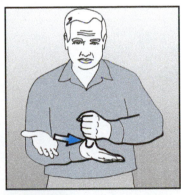

CUT-OFF

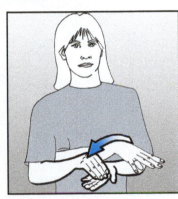

COPY

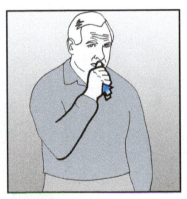

SECRET

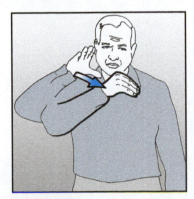

SHUT-UP

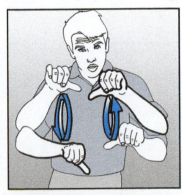

CHEMICAL, medicine

24

English Translations of Dialogues

(Please note that other translations may also be possible.)

UNIT 1 *Introductions and Personal Information*

Introductions

Alex: I don't know you. What's your name?
Lisa: My name is Lisa Benes. What's your name?
Alex: My name is Alex Jones. It's nice to meet you.
Lisa: It's nice to meet you.

Personal information

Alex: Are you a student?
Lisa: Yes, I'm a student. You?
Alex: No, I'm not a student.
Lisa: Are you Deaf?
Alex: Yes, I'm Deaf. Are you hearing?
Lisa: Yes, I'm hearing.

More personal information

Lisa: Where are you from?
Alex: I'm from New York.
Lisa: I'm from California
Alex: Where do you live?
Lisa: I live in San Diego. Are you a student?
Alex: No. I'm your teacher.

UNIT 2 *Learning ASL*

Going to class

Chris: Are you taking an ASL class?
Lisa: Yes, I'm taking one.
Chris: Which class?
Lisa: The class is "ASL 1."
Chris: Me, too! Where is the class?
Lisa: The class is at the college.

Objects in the classroom

Chris: Do you have a pencil?
Lisa: Yes, I have one. Where's the paper?
Chris: The paper is over there. Do you have the book?
Lisa: No, where is the book?

335

Showing you understand and asking for help

Alex: Do you understand?
Lisa: I don't understand. Please repeat.
Alex: This class is "ASL 1."
Lisa: Oh, I understand.

UNIT 3 *Politeness*

Asking politely

Lisa: Excuse me. Where's the library?
Alex: I'm going in that direction now. Come with me.
Lisa: Fine. Wait a minute please. I'll get my book.
Alex: Okay. I'm not in a hurry.

Thanks

Pat: Can you help me out?
Chris: Sure, what do you need?
Pat: Thank you. I need to bring a box here.
Chris: Sure, where is the box?
Pat: Thanks very much.

Interruptions and apologies

Lisa Excuse me.
Pat: What?
Lisa: I'm sorry. Where is the restroom?
Pat: Down there.
Lisa: Thank you.

UNIT 4 *Descriptions*

Physical appearance

Chris: Do you know my teacher?
Pat: No, I don't. What does she look like?
Chris: Her hair is shoulder-length and black, and her eyes are brown.
Pat: Tell me more.
Chris: She's tall and thin.
Pat: Oh, I know who she is.

Clothing

Pat: Do you know the woman in the red dress?
Alex: Which one?
Pat: The one with vertical stripes and a long skirt.
Alex: You mean the one with the white hat?
Pat: That's the one.

Personality and Character

Chris: See that man with the beard, he's nice. Do you know him?
Alex: I haven't met him.
Chris: He's friendly. That man, he's arrogant.
Alex: I know him. You're right. He's arrogant.

UNIT 5 *Requests*

Polite commands

(Several people are in a room.)
Alex: Please flash the lights.
(Lisa flashes the lights on and off.)
Alex: Close the door. It feels a little cold.
(Lisa closes the door.)
Alex: Thank you. Please sit down.
(Everyone sits down.)
Alex: Now, let's get started.

Requests to do something

Lisa: Would you mind opening the window?
Chris: Sure!
Lisa: Thanks. And can you do one more thing?
Chris: What?
Lisa: Can you throw out the garbage?
Chris: Okay. You owe me one.

More requests

Chris: Please turn on the TV.
(Lisa turns on the TV.)
(Later.)
Chris: Please turn on the light. I can't see.
(Lisa turns on the light.)
(Later phone lights flash.)
Chris: Please answer that for me.
Lisa: Wait a minute! I'm tired of this. Do it yourself!

UNIT 6 *Expressing Yourself*

How you feel

Pat: Good morning! How are you?
Alex: I'm so-so. How're you?
Pat: I'm fine. What's wrong?
Alex: I tossed and turned all night. I'm tired.
Pat: Oh. I'm sorry. Do you want some coffee?
Alex: Yes!

Opinions and preferences

Lisa: Wow. You look mad. What's wrong?
Pat: John didn't show up.
Lisa: Oh. Is he late?
Pat: Yes. I don't like it.
Lisa: I'm not surprised.

Anxiety

Lisa: I'm nervous.
Chris: Stop worrying!
Lisa: I must pass this test.
Chris: You'll pass. Calm down.
Lisa   I'll flunk.

UNIT 7 *More Descriptions*

Objects and their location

Chris: I put my glass there. Now it's gone.
Lisa: I took the glass to the kitchen.
Chris: Where did you put it?
Lisa: I put it on the table.

Objects, number, and location

Chris: I put the apples there, don't touch them.
Lisa: You'd better hide them.
Chris: No. I'm going to leave them there. Don't touch them.

How many

Lisa: Do you have any clothes? I'm going to do some washing.
Chris: Yes. I have some. I'll bring them.
(Chris brings a pile of clothes.)
Lisa: Wow! That's a lot of shirts. How many are there?
Chris: I think eight. And four pairs of pants.
Lisa: It looks like you haven't washed clothes for a month.

UNIT 8 *Family and Friends*

Family information

Alex: My family is having a reunion tomorrow. We haven't gotten together for two years.
Chris: Is your family Deaf?
Alex: My parents are Deaf. My sister is Deaf. I have two brothers, one is Deaf, the other is hearing.
Chris: Does your hearing brother sign?
Alex: Of course!

Family relationships

Alex: Yesterday I met your husband. How long have you two been married?
Pat: We've been married for six years.
Alex: Wow! I didn't realize it's been a long time. Do you have children?
Pat: Two daughters and a son.
Alex: Are they Deaf or hearing?
Pat: All are Deaf.

Friends and acquaintances

Chris: I saw you yesterday. Were you with a friend?
Lisa: He's a close friend. We grew up together.
Chris: Is he your boyfriend?
Lisa: (gestures, no) We're just friends.
Chris: Oh. It looked like you were going together. I was mistaken.

UNIT 9 *More Descriptions*

How others look

Pat: Do you see that woman there? She's beautiful.
Lisa: Do you know her?
Pat: No. I don't know her.
Lisa: You know her. That's Maria.
Pat: Really! That one. I saw her when she was five years old. She was short and chubby. Now she's changed. I'm stunned.

Personality

Alex: John was stubborn.
Pat: I know. I remember when we were little at the school for the Deaf. On weekends John didn't want to go home. He wanted to stay at the school. His parents pulled him by the arm. He was stubborn and wouldn't go. His parents would give up. John stayed and played. He was extremely mischievous.
Alex: He's still mischievous.

Physical features

Lisa: I'm looking for a man, I forgot his name. He is tall, wears glasses, and has a potbelly. Do you know him?
Pat: I don't know who you mean.
Lisa: He has broad shoulders and a mustache.
Pat: Oh. I think he already left.
Lisa: Oh, gee!

UNIT 10 *At Home and Daily Living*

Your residence

Alex: I recently moved to a new house. It has three bedrooms, two baths, a living room, and kitchen. I like it.

Pat: Did you move the furniture yourself?

Alex: Yes. I borrowed a truck. I backed it up, loaded it, and drove to the new house and unloaded. When I was finished, I was exhausted.

Objects in your residence

Alex: My house is new and big with two floors. It has bedrooms upstairs and a basement downstairs. It has a dining room with a big square window. In the dining room is a big square table that is pretty when the sun shines on it.

Pat: Do you have a family room?

Alex: Yes. It's my favorite. It has a long sofa in front of a TV. I sit there and watch TV.

Pat: Wow, that's nice.

What you do every day

Chris: Now that you've retired, what do you do everyday?

Pat: I enjoy taking it easy. Every morning I get up, read the newspaper and drink coffee. I don't usually eat breakfast. Most of the time I go out to lunch. Every night I cook. Sometimes I get a movie and put it in my DVD player and watch it.

Chris: What do you do on weekends?

Pat: Saturdays I clean up the house and wash clothes. Sundays I go for a walk and rest in the afternoon.

UNIT 11 *Food and Food Shopping*

The menu

Lisa: What do you want to do tonight?

Chris: I'll cook something. I think vegetable soup, chicken, potatoes and a salad, that's all. And some ice cream.

Lisa: Fine. Something easy.

Chris: I thought of something. We're out of potatoes and oil. I can't go to the store. I don't have the time. Do you mind going?

Lisa: I don't mind.

Quantities

Lisa: I'll show you how to make a pie.

Chris: What kind of pie?

Lisa: Coconut. First, we need two eggs.

Chris: I bought a dozen.

Lisa: Fine. We need half a pound of butter, a cup of milk, a cup of sugar.

Chris: Will you make a thin or thick pie?

Lisa: Watch me and I'll show you.

Prices

Chris: I'm shocked. I went to the store. The prices are way up.

Lisa: What did you buy?

Chris: I bought three apples. They cost $2.00. A pound of butter cost $3.99 and a gallon of ice cream cost four something.

Lisa: Wow, that's expensive. What was the total?

Chris: I went to the store with $50 and came home with 50 cents left.

Lisa: That's awful.

UNIT 12 *Offering and Declining*

Food and drink

Pat: Do you want something to eat?

Alex: Sure. I haven't eaten all day. I'm hungry.

Pat: I'm making a sandwich. Do you want one?

Alex: Fine, anything.

Pat: What do you want to drink? There's beer, coke, water.

Alex: Coke, thank you. Would you like some help?

Offering help

Alex: Can I use the TTY to call my brother? My car won't start. I've tried everything and I give up.

Pat: Is something wrong with the motor?

Alex: I'm not sure. It has gas. Maybe the battery is dead.

Pat: How old is the battery?

Alex: Four years.

Pat: I suspect it is dead. Do you want me to jump it for you?

Declining and explaining

Chris: I can't make it to your party. I have a conflict.

Alex: All right. I'll save some food for you.

Chris: No. I'm gaining weight. I just thought of something. I'm supposed to bring a salad. What should I do?

Alex: Don't worry about it. I'll do it myself.

Chris: Thanks. Will you tell your wife I'm sorry?

Alex: Sure. It's okay, don't worry.

UNIT 13 *More Ways to Express Yourself*

Satisfaction and dissatisfaction

Pat: Come and look at this door. It's not right. You have to do it over.

Chris: Why? What's wrong?

Pat: See the edges around the door. It's sloppy. I'm not satisfied.

Chris: Do I have to do it over?

Pat: Yes, you must. Just good enough is not acceptable to me. It must be exact.

Agreement and disagreement

Lisa: I don't agree that the three of us should look for a house.

Chris: What? I thought we agreed. Do you have a different idea?

Lisa: My idea was to take the money and give it to her and she would decide, not all of us.

Chris: I think differently. I want to see it first. If I'm satisfied, I'll pay.

Lisa: I disagree.

Chris: What do we do?

Concern and feelings

Pat: Are you all right? You look sad. Someone told me your dog passed away. Is that true?

Chris: Yes, I feel down.

Pat: I'm sorry. Do you plan to get another?

Chris: I don't know. I miss my dog. Replacing him will be hard. I don't know.

Pat: That's too bad. Come with me for a bike ride, maybe you'll feel better.

Chris: Thanks. I'm alright. You go ahead.

UNIT 14 *Experiences and Current Activity*

An event

Pat: I decided to go see a movie. When I arrived, there were scads of cars. I drove around for 15 minutes and couldn't park. Finally a car pulled out and I parked. I went to buy a ticket and there was a long line of people. Finally I got in the theater and sat down. Then it hit me, my car lights, did I turn them off? I couldn't remember. I watched the movie until it was over, then ran to my car. Of course the battery was dead.

A past event

Chris: Yesterday I was playing softball and when I was up to bat I was hit in the eye by a ball. Wow! My eye hurt. It swelled up.

Alex: Wow! That happened to me before. I was hit in the eye and it swelled up like yours.

Chris: What happened?

Alex: Two years ago while I was driving, I had an accident and was hit in the eye.

Current activity

Lisa: What's up?

Chris: I'm taking out these old cabinets and putting in new ones.

Lisa: I didn't know you were good at woodwork. Where did you learn?

Chris: At the school for the Deaf. Now I'm putting a round edge on the door.

Lisa: Wow! You're good.

Chris: If you have the right machines, it's easy.

UNIT 15 *Future Plans and Obligations*

General future plans

Lisa: When I graduate from high school, I'm going to college.

Chris: I don't want to go to college.

Lisa: After graduation, what will you do?

Chris: I want an easy, regular job. I don't want stress.

Lisa: Will you get married and have children?

Chris: I don't know. I'm thinking about it.

Time and place to meet

Alex: What time should I pick you up next week?

Pat: You mean to go to Los Angeles?

Alex: Yes, what time?

Pat: At eight in the morning. Okay?

Alex: Fine. I'll meet you at your house and you can join me in my car.

Pat: Okay, I'll wait outside in front.

Alex: If traffic's bad, I might be late. Be patient and wait. I'll show up.

Future obligations

Chris: Let's go swimming.

Alex: I can't. I have a doctor's appointment at 2 o'clock.

Chris: Oh. Tomorrow night can you come to my house and we'll watch a captioned DVD?

Alex: No, I have to work at the club.

Chris: Wow! You're so busy. I should have made an appointment with you two months ago.

UNIT 16 *Directions and Instructions*

Directions

Pat: Excuse me. Is there a drug store nearby?

Alex: Yes. You go out, turn left, drive to the intersection, then turn left. You go straight ahead through two intersections and it's on the corner.

Pat: How do I go out?

Alex: Oh. You haven't been here before?

Pat: No, never.

Alex: Okay. Take the elevator down to the first floor, turn right, and there's the exit.

Descriptions of places

Chris: Do you want to go to Jose's restaurant?

Lisa: I don't know where it is.

Chris: You know the building with the white front and green roof. There's a sign that says "Jose's."

Lisa: I don't know it. What's it near?

Chris: The temple is here and the restaurant is here.

Instructions

Alex: You have to be careful. The computer is expensive and breaks easy.

Lisa: Okay, I'm not a kid.

Alex: Okay. Open the box. Take it out and put it on the table. Find the book. Follow that book! Look for the cord and plug it in. Look for a disk and put it in. When you're finished, turn it on. Wait until the screen lights up, and then it's ready.

UNIT 17 *Suggestions and Advice*

Suggestions

Chris: I'm bored. What do you want to do tonight?

Lisa: I have two suggestions, you choose. My first suggestion is that we go bowling. Tonight is Deaf bowling night.

Chris: Okay, what's the other thing?

Lisa: If you don't want to go bowling, why don't we go to a movie.

Chris: I'm tired of going bowling every week. Let's go to a movie.

Time and place

Pat: Do you want to meet again?

Lisa: Fine. When?

Pat: Next week on Friday?

Lisa: Fine. What time?

Pat: Nine in the morning?

Lisa: Better make it around eleven. At your house, right?

Pat: Right.

Advice

Pat: The money hasn't come. What should I do?

Chris: Did you TTY her?

Pat: I paged her on Monday. She told me I would get it today. Should I call her again?

Chris: Better not. Maybe you should get a lawyer.

Pat: Should I tell her I will get a lawyer, or...?

Chris: Better not say anything. Ask the lawyer.

UNIT 18 *Attitudes and Opinions*

What others think

Lisa: Let me ask you. Do you think the food here is good?

Alex: Why are you asking me?

Lisa: You two come here often, right?

Alex: Right. Why do you want to know?

Lisa: I'm writing an article for the college newspaper.

Alex: Will you use our names?

Lisa: No names. Okay? Do you like the food here?

Opinions

Lisa: That's odd. I made a pizza and it tastes lousy.

Chris: Why? What's wrong with it?

Lisa: I don't know. Taste it.

(Chris tastes it.)

Chris: It's delicious!

Lisa: No! It tastes awful.

Chris: I think it's fine.

Values

Pat: I don't believe in large families with several children.

Lisa: I want a lot of children. Why are you against that?

Pat: The world already has too many children. I support adoption.

Lisa: I don't mind adoption if I can have one or two of my own. Do you accept that?

Pat: I accept that. I believe we must take care of the children.

Lisa: Right. I agree 100 percent.

UNIT 19 *Recreational Activities*

Activities

Alex: Do you like to ski?

Pat: I love it. I go there often in the winter.

Alex: Where do you like to go?

Pat: To Big Bear. It's nearby. I can drive there easily.

Alex: Is there a lot of snow?

Pat: Yes, a lot. It's nice. Not a lot of people.

Alex: If you go, can I join you?

Pat: Sure.

A sequence of activities

Alex: What did you do last weekend?

Chris: A group of us went to the beach. We went early and got a place and set up for volleyball. We played for two hours and then we went for a swim. We cooked hot dogs and hamburgers and ate a lot. After that we lay in the sun and went to sleep. Later we woke up and went swimming. Then we played frisbee. When it got dark, we lit a fire and we sat in a circle and talked.

Alex: Wow! Fun!

Seasonal activities

Pat: I can't wait for fall when the trees will change color. I'm going to the mountains and walk through the trees.

Lisa: Me, too. I'm going to go camping.

Pat: I have one complaint, fall seems short. In one or two weeks it's over.

Lisa: True, but I like snow. I can cross-country ski.

Pat: True, that's fun. Do you play basketball?

Lisa: Sometimes. If I join a team, I will play.

UNIT 20 *Travel—Places and Experiences*

Travel experience

Lisa: Two weeks ago I drove to Washington. My parents wanted to come with me. I said okay. They were excited. We left Tuesday morning with no problem. Later we stopped for lunch. Mom always reminds Dad to take his pill. Mom worries a lot about Dad's heart. Dad doesn't want to take the pills. If Mom keeps reminding him, Dad hates it. I knew that my parents tend to quarrel. I was repeatedly embarrassed. Finally they were quiet. From then on it was okay.

Alex: Were you relieved?

Lisa: (emphatic) Yes!

More travel experiences

Alex: I'll never forget going to Europe. I traveled for two months.

Pat: Did you travel alone?

Alex: Yes. I got around on the train. I met Deaf people several times.

Pat: Wow! Wish I had gone with you. Did the trip go smoothly?

Alex: Yes. A friend of mine told me she was continually frustrated trying to find a place to sleep. I was continually worried, but I found I had no problem.

Places you visited

Alex: I went to Holland and visited a flower place. Have you been there?

Pat: No. I've heard that Holland has scads of flowers.

Alex: Right. Holland is very wet, so it's easy to grow them. Anyway, one place, I don't know the name, sells flowers. I was very impressed. I went in a building and could see flowers all over. In loud colors. It was strange because it was fall and very cold outside. Where were the flowers from, I wonder?

UNIT 21 *Occupations and Professions*

Occupations and professions

Alex: What work do you do?

Chris: I'm a welder. I have worked for a shipbuilder for two years.

Alex: Oh. I didn't realize that. I thought you worked at the post office, I was wrong.

Chris: I never worked at the post office. A long time ago I was a mechanic. I switched to welding because it pays better money. What do you do?

Alex: I teach ASL and I'm a painter.

Chris: What do you paint?

Alex: Houses, buildings, bridges, anything.

Job activity

Pat: You work in a bank right?

Lisa: Right.

Pat: What do you do exactly?

Lisa: I do computer input. I feed info from checks and deposit slips into the computer. I'm a supervisor, I have three people under me. If a problem comes up, I help solve it.

Pat: Do you work days?

Lisa: Yes. I work a 4 day week. But ten hours straight then I'm off for 3 days.

Pat: Oh. That's a great idea.

Work history

Alex: What do you do?

Pat: I'm retired.

Alex: Oh. You look young. What did you do before?

Pat: Different things. First I worked as a painter. I didn't like it so I quit. I applied for a job as a printer with the Washington *Post*. I worked for six years and was laid off and moved to Los Angeles. I looked for a job but couldn't find one so I got unemployment insurance. Later I was hired by the L.A. *Times*. I worked nights for 30 years. Now I'm retired.

UNIT 22 *The Body, Health, and Emergencies*

Physical conditioning

Chris: Wow! You look good. Have you been exercising?

Lisa: Yes. Everyday I run about 3 or 4 miles.

Chris: I'm impressed. I often go to the spa to lift weights.

Lisa: Do you lift weights with your legs?

Chris: Yes. Also I do knee bends with weights on my shoulders.

Lisa: Do you want to run with me?

Chris: No, I'm bored with running.

Health and health problems

Lisa: I heard you were in the hospital. What happened?

Alex: Yes. I almost had a heart attack. It wasn't bad. I'm fine.

Lisa: Oh. I didn't know. How did it happen?

Alex: I've been under stress and got no exercise and ate too much. I was working and felt chest pains for two or three days. I decided to go to a doctor. The doctor examined me and took my blood pressure. Wow! It was high. He immediately put me in the hospital. I had to lie calmly in bed and takes pills for one week. After than I went home and couldn't work for two months. I'm well now. My blood pressure is normal.

Emergencies

Alex: A man just fell down and seems sick. Someone must call 911 to call an ambulance.

Chris: Ask that woman, she can hear.

Alex: You go cover him up and keep him warm.

(later)

Chris: Did you get through? Is an ambulance coming?

Alex: Yes. I wrote a note to the woman. She understood and called. It should arrive in five minutes.

Chris: He seems to be breathing okay. I wonder if he fainted?

Alex: I don't know. I have never experienced this before.

UNIT 23 *Current Events*

Recent news

Alex: Have you heard?

Pat: What?

Alex: There was an earthquake in California near L.A. Some building walls cracked and roofs fell in.

Pat: How did you find out? When did it happen?

Alex: This morning. I just saw the news on TV.

Pat: In exactly what part of L.A.?

Alex: It seemed to be in the southeast.

Pat: My son lives in L.A. I should call to check.

Current topics of interest

Chris: I liked that movie we saw yesterday.

Lisa: I liked it too. I want to see it again.

Chris: Yes. The movie was different, it's hard to explain.

Lisa: What do you mean?

Chris: It's hard to explain. It looked different, the color was different, dark. There was no sun in the movie. It made me feel involved. It made me depressed, scared, and my heart would jump. You didn't know what would happen.

Lisa: Right, but some of the characters were not real and were exaggerated.

Chris: But some were perfect, like the little brother.

Lisa: Yes. It was a good movie.

Current issues

Lisa: Poverty is the worst problem. All countries have it. I understand poor countries having poor people. But what's worse is that there are poor people here in the United States. I don't understand that.

Pat: Right. Here in the U.S. many people have money.

Lisa: Many people who are poor, it's not their fault. Some can't work due to health problems. Some can work but don't have the right skills. Many are too old to work. The government gives some support but not enough. What can we do?

Pat: You're asking me? I don't know the answer either.

UNIT 24 *How Things Are Done*

A process

Lisa: Something's wrong. This machine doesn't work. What should I do?

Alex: What happened?

Lisa: The paper was running through the machine fine, then it stopped.

Alex: Let me look. Oh. That light means paper is jammed inside. You have to open the machine and pull out this tray and take out the paper.

Lisa: You take out the paper, I'm clumsy.

Alex: No. You have to learn. Take it out yourself.

Width, length, and height

Chris: I want to show you a table I made.

Pat: You made a dining table?

Chris: Yes. I made the table top. The length is 72 inches. The width is 36 inches.

Pat: How did you make it?

Chris: I put two pieces of flat wood together. I measured and cut the legs. I wanted the table to be 30 inches high.

Pat: How did you know the measurements?

Chris: I copied them from another table.

Measurements and weight

Lisa: Wow! That's a lot of Christmas presents. What's in this box?

Chris: It's a secret. No, it's not a secret. It's a new TV.

Lisa: Wow! What's the diagonal measurement?

Chris: 19 inches.

Lisa: That's nice. What's in this box?

Chris: It's candy for grandma.

Lisa: Wow! It's heavy. How much does it weigh?

Chris: 3 pounds.

Lisa: How much does grandma weigh?

Chris: Stop fooling around.

Vocabulary Index

Note: Entries in upper case are vocabulary words; those in lower case are secondary meanings of vocabulary words; those in italics are conceptual entries.